The Mental and Physical Way to a...

# Younger Body Now

By Arthur Driscoll Jr. and
Arthur Driscoll III

With contributions by Nancy Driscoll
Author, Every Mind Matters

# Acknowledgements

I want to thank my brother John who believed we could write a great book and encouraged us to get started, his wife Nancy who helped research and prepare the book for publication, our clients who inspire us daily, and our family for encouraging my son and I to share our story in order to inspire others - young and old - to a life of health and fitness.

I also want to thank Eric Slayton, owner of New York Underground Fitness where we train our clients and filmed the workout portion of the DVDs; Lyle Schuler, owner of MAC Fitness in Kingston, New York, where we filmed the testimonials and workouts with our clients; and also my daughter Kayla who flew in from Georgia to take part in the shooting of the workout DVDs. My son wants to thank his high school track coach from Onteora High School, Mike Boms, for instilling in him that education is the most important thing - track is icing on the cake.

**Visit Us On The Web**

**www.youngerbodybyart.com**

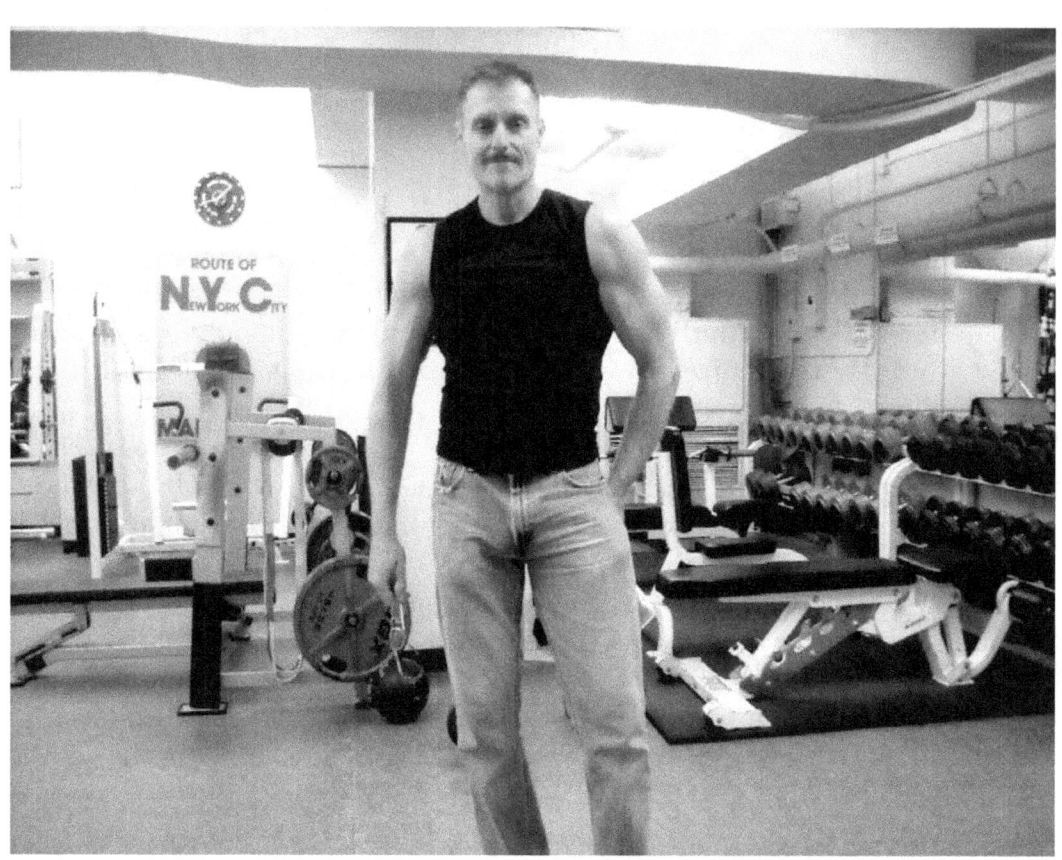

*You really are as young as you feel!*

## About the author...

Art Driscoll has been a fitness professional for 25 years, devoting his life to training and coaching others. Being involved in the health and fitness fields since the industry got started, he has an enormous amount of knowledge to not only keep himself in shape but to keep others fit as well. He has competed in a wide variety of sports: track and field, mountain biking, and cycling. As a nationally-competitive bodybuilder he finished second place in the ANPPC-USA Body Building Championships, and also completed many triathlons, biathlons and marathons. This has helped him coach and train a wide variety of athletes and clients ranging from high school and college athletes to people well into their 80s. He was a personal trainer before personal training was part of the fitness industry. Owning a number of fitness centers has further developed his ability to train clients on every level. He was featured on CNBC demonstrating with his clients, especially women over 60, what can be achieved with proper training principles. Today he still runs with the college athletes he trains and once a year competes in a bodybuilding show to keep his edge.

His knowledge of nutrition comes from his 25 years of experience in the fitness field, allowing him to give his clients the best nutritional advice for maximum health and fitness. Having to diet for numerous bodybuilding shows and athletic events has enabled him to pass on to his clients who want to lose weight and get healthy, the hands-on knowledge that made him a success. The many success stories from the clients he has trained are a testament to his knowledge and ability. Anyone that follows his principles can be successful in their fitness goals and achieve a younger body now!

## About The Co-Author...

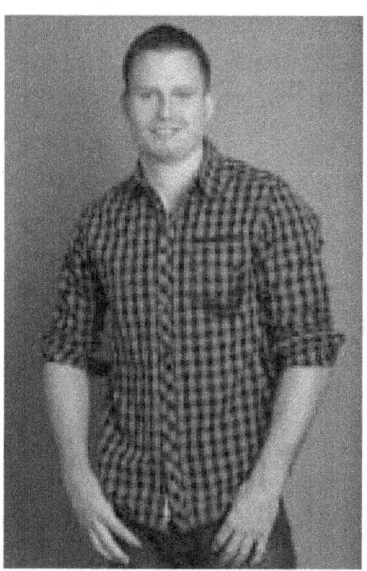

Art Driscoll III, co-author of "Younger Body Now", brings a broader approach to the book's strength training and cardio routines. By combining old school with new school training philosophies, father and son provide clients a unique way to approach the workouts. Being brought up in an atmosphere of participating and competing in a wide variety of sports, Art got interested in the health and fitness field at an early age. Activities such as rock climbing, skiing, snowboarding, and mountain biking helped him develop into a competitive athlete.

Art began competing in cycling and mountain bike races and by the time he was 14 years old he raced in the junior sport division in the Norba USA National Mountain Bike Championship. In high school he competed in cross country and track and became the Conference and Section 9 Champion in the 200- and 400-meter sprints, setting school records in the 300- and 400-meters. In college he became an All-

American in track by running on the 4 by 400 relay team in the National Championships. Growing up he spent much of his time in his father's gyms and fitness centers observing and learning the fitness industry.  After college he studied to become a Certified Personal Trainer and received two certifications in the fitness field.  After working at a major fitness center he started his own business as an independent personal trainer.

Art was very instrumental in making the "Younger Body Now" DVDs. He not only helped to organize and write the script for the DVDs, which included the testimonials and work-outs, but participated in them as well.  Having knowledge and experience in the fitness field well beyond his years, he has added important information for the reader of "Younger Body Now".

As Art himself notes: "I've had many challenges in my life that my dad and I have gone through together.  From rock climbing the toughest climbs, to riding up the steepest hills in mountain bike races, I thrive on challenge.  When my dad came to me and asked me to take on a new challenge of helping write the book, 'Younger Body Now,' I jumped at the opportunity.  Being involved in writing the book and making and filming the DVDs have been great experiences for me.  Seeing the amazing results my dad and I have gotten with our clients over the years was motivation enough to work on the project.

I was fortunate enough to compete in a wide variety of sports my whole life and learned that to become a great athlete you need the proper mindset.  My dad taught me to use my mind to beat my competition, and today I teach my clients how to use their minds to get the results they want too. It's been a long journey since my dad first asked me to help write 'Younger Body Now'. Seeing a finished product that we are both so proud of has been fulfilling for the both of us."

Since I've been doing the 30-minute workout my quality of life has increased significantly. It is the best thing I could have done for myself. I feel and look great!

Gail Postal, 63

# Contents

I've been working out for years, but since I started doing the 30-minute workouts I've put on ten pounds of muscle and I'm twice as strong with more endurance.  It's the best favor you can do for yourself!

Ted Faraone, 53

# Younger Body Now Introduction

It took me twenty-five years to write this book –Younger Body Now. Twenty-five years of learning, observing, studying, training hundreds of people, opening and closing my own gyms, and competing in a wide variety of sports.   It took being part of an industry that started in a comic book with some big bully kicking sand in a poor, skinny wimp's face. After doing his Charles Atlas routines the guy comes back to get revenge on the bully and win the girl. The fitness industry has come a long way since then, evolving into a multi-million dollar industry.

Being part of this evolution has been a great experience for me. I wanted to share what I have learned with anyone who is willing to listen, in as short and simple a way as possible.

Although growing old can be a terrible experience, it doesn't have to be that way. We can grow old gracefully and keep ourselves as young as possible for as long we can, or we can have aches and pains and health problems. The choice is ours but optimum health is not a gift - it takes work. I have chosen to keep my body young and super fit. What a rewarding feeling it is now to see my clients reverse the aging process and get stronger and fitter as the years go by as well.

Yes, the fitness field has come a long way since I was a young boy reading my favorite comic books. Now it's your turn to start reversing your body age and feeling younger right now. This book is dedicated to all the people I have trained for without them this experiment in growing older but feeling younger would not have been possible.

I used to be a model and since I retired I've managed to maintain my body weight and athletic look with Art's workouts.

...Heather Cooksey, 32

## *1*

# You Really Are As Young As You Feel!

## The Factors Involved In Aging

Many factors – physiological, sociological, psychological - are involved in the process of aging. There are inevitable physical changes in the body as we age.  Sociological factors include changes in work life or retirement, society's views and biases about age, family and financial challenges, etc.

A critical aspect of the psychological factor however is that we often begin to lower our expectations of what we think we should be able to do. Because actions follow thinking, our lifestyles begin to change to reflect our changed beliefs.

We assume aches and pains are normal because everyone we know seems to have them. We see ourselves in commercials buying arthritis medicine, "silver formula" vitamins, and other pills for all the problems we must surely be having –at our age. We doze off in front of the TV and talk at work about how tired we always are.  We wonder why we don't feel as steady as we used to, wondering if we are developing some dread disease. Someone reminds us we "aren't a kid anymore" and we resign ourselves to a life of reduced vitality and energy. We believe we should slow down - so we do. The less active we become the more tired we get and this becomes the self-fulfilling prophecy.  Our minds still think great thoughts but our bodies just don't seem to want to respond.

## Physiological Changes

Of course there are real physiological changes going on as we age. The body convinces the mind to slow down and the more we slow down the greater the physiological effects of aging become. As we become more sedentary we lose muscle, our endurance weakens, we become less flexible, and our energy levels are further depleted. All these physiological changes provide a domino effect that makes us even more inactive. Who wants to exercise when you are tired and aching already?

*Our minds still think great thoughts but our bodies just don't seem to want to respond.*

Being inactive also slows down our metabolism and we begin to gain weight. This in turn has another psychological effect – an impact on our vanity. We don't want to look in the mirror because we don't like what we see yet we are too tired to do anything about it.

To make matters worse, this excessive weight gain and loss of energy, muscle, bone density, and overall lack of physical well-being and fitness relate to all the talked-about degenerative diseases that plague us as we get older. These include high blood pressure, arthritis, heart disease, diabetes and obesity to name a few.  Put this package together and we can feel old – really – old.

Clearly we all live very different life styles. Still what we have in common is that those lifestyles are usually fast-paced and high-stress. Whether you're a personal trainer and body builder in New York City like I am, a teacher in suburban Maryland, a computer consultant in Texas, or a construction worker in Chicago, it's hard to find the time to exercise, eat better, and focus on your health.

*We'd like our bodies to keep up with our minds, but those bodies just aren't cooperating like they did 10, 20, or 30 years ago.*

In my long career as a personal trainer, I have dealt with people in all walks of life, at all ages and fitness levels, and varying levels of initial motivation. After twenty five years in the health and personal fitness business I have found that most people have a very hard time getting started on the path to better health, even once they make the commitment to work out.

Even though we don't feel well, our clothes don't fit, we can't do things we used to, and we all complain about our latest body crisis, we just don't believe that anything can be done.  We'd like our bodies to keep up with our minds, but those bodies just aren't cooperating like they did 10, 20, or 30 years ago.

Even with the best intentions, doctor's orders, and spouses' gentle encouragement, we put things off until days turn into months and months turn into years. In reality can we really reverse the aging process and turn back the clock to start feeling younger? Can we really start to feel as good as we used to? Can we do something about the onset of chronic disease or minimize its impact? The answer is YES and you can start today!

Of course everyone is different and will have different results. Based on specific physical limitations, age, the level of effort and time commitment, eating habits, genetics, the presence of any chronic health conditions, and the type of program chosen – results can and will vary. Someone who is sixty, has been very inactive, and has chronic health problems will certainly have a greater challenge than someone who is 50, reasonably active, and in overall good health.

**Still everyone – *yes everyone* – can have a Younger Body Now.**

## Mind Over Muscle

Mental outlook is a key place to start to turn back the body's aging process. You can only do what you think you can do. Through experience I have found that feeling younger starts in your mind. If you place no limits on what you believe you can accomplish, no matter how old you are you will see results – guaranteed. It's harder to train a young athlete with a negative mindset than to work with an older client who has a positive mental outlook. It really is your mind that matters in the fitness business.

## It's your mind that matters in the fitness business!

One thing is for certain. Once anyone starts to exercise – *starts to do any exercise at all* - their body will respond and they will feel younger immediately.

Not all exercises are the same just as not all trainers are the same although each offers his or her own "claim to fame". It took me years of trial and error and experimentation to find out what type of exercise is the best, at what duration, and at what intensity, for peak results. With my son adding the latest training techniques and exercises, we developed the routines used in this book for maximum results in the shortest amount of time. The bottom line is that any exercise that keeps you moving is better than nothing, and doing it "*now*" is much better than doing it "*later*"!

*The harder you work, the better the results!*

Through scientific studies in the areas of sports medicine and aging we now know that the harder you work out the better the results. You burn more calories, your conditioning improves, the heart becomes stronger, and you build muscle and lose weight faster. There are basically some broad types of exercise that are typically recommended: cardio workouts, individual or team sports, and strength training.

## The Importance of Cardio

In cardio, you have several options including walking, running – either on a treadmill or outside – use of gym equipment from stair masters to elliptical machines, biking, swimming, and hiking. Many of us join gyms with the best intention of getting our hearts pumping again. Recommendations are for adults to get at least thirty minutes of cardio workouts several times per week. We are even encouraged to take a walk at lunch or take the stairs instead of the elevator at work.

*Feeling like the "glory days" are over?*

## Sports Exercise

Many of us engaged in sports when we were younger. These included fast-paced team sports such as football, baseball, and basketball or more individualized sports such as tennis, martial arts, track and field, or golf.  Some of us still try a pick-up game of football or basketball on Sunday afternoon only to find we are too out of shape to score a point. We think those "glory days" are over and the best place to enjoy our favorite sport is from the couch. Won't it really require long hours at the gym or on the tread mill to improve our fitness? Who wants to do that?  Who has the time?

Years ago there was a Swedish study which indicated that longer, lower levels of intense cardio were the best for burning fat and getting fit. Being a track athlete, coach, and trainer, I knew that didn't make sense.  The best-trained athletes of all the sport participants I observed were definitely track sprinters.

## Sprinters Show Us The Way

Sprinters train at a high level of intensity with short, fast interval training which gives them great overall fitness and great bodies as well. Of course someone who is training to run a longer distance such as the mile or a marathon has to train differently to build endurance for that type of event. Still for those of us who want to burn body fat, build strength, and increase our metabolism —and spend as little time as possible doing it - short and intense workouts are the key to success. That's why the regimen I recommend teaches short, intense, workouts.

The latest studies have proven what seemed obvious to me all along. Short, intense exercise is much more beneficial than long, lower intensity workouts. A short period of intense exercise burns more fat and calories than a lower intensity exercise over a longer period of time. It also speeds up your metabolism so you are actually still burning calories hours after you stop exercising. This same theory goes with any exercise routine. Shorter, more intense routines are much better and time efficient than a longer, slower routine for overall fitness.

## Weight Training Is The Key

So what then is the best form of exercise for reversing body age to start feeling younger? Regular cardio exercises are critical. The latest studies also indicate that weight training is a key component to overall fitness and improving body age. Weight training or strength training works on all the areas that begin to diminish when we age: muscle mass and strength, bone density, core strength, flexibility, and tendon and ligament strength. Nothing does more for increasing overall body strength in the legs and upper body than weight training.

There are many types of weight training: circuit training, body building, power lifting, etc. As for which one is the best and where to start the answer is to do a *combination of each* and develop this combination into a routine like my son and I have done in the workouts in this book.

A 30-minute workout combines all the different types of weight training into one routine. We have assembled the top three personal training components we could find and developed a system that has proven itself over and over. With over 25 years of experience I have shown that anyone - aged 30 - 80 - can start feeling younger and keep that younger body age indefinitely. I have selected people that have benefited from my methods to share their stories and tell you themselves what results they achieved.

With our training plan I can take a 50-, 60-, or even 70-year-old and help them do things most people half their age cannot do. A couple of years ago I had a 72-year-old woman named Judy Milstein leg press 1000 pounds on national TV, showing that her bone density and muscle strength were far superior to anyone her age. She was not an exception!  I have trained many men and women to do extraordinary things -  building their strength, fitness, and endurance levels -  by using my program.

Just recently two of my 54-year-old female clients, Margaret Clemons, and Sophia Stanika, competed in the 2009 American Masters Weightlifting Championships.  Neither were ever competitive athletes and both have been training with me for two years with the 30-minute short, intense workout.  They had gotten in very good shape and were fairly strong from our workouts.  I asked them both if they wanted to take their fitness a step further and train for the two Olympic lifts; the snatch and the clean and jerk.  Olympic lifting is a very technical sport that requires speed, strength, and agility.  After only a year of training, they won first and second place medals in their weight classes.  Their accomplishment was a testimonial that if you work out hard and have the right mental attitude and the right coaching, you will succeed.

"I'm 41 years old and I don't have time to spend hours in the gym getting in shape. Only twice a week with the short intense workout, I'm in the best shape of my life. I can work longer hours, have more energy, and I can spend more quality time with my kids."

Steve Chaikelson

## 2

# A Little History Sets the Stage

## Weight Lifting In The Olympics

In the late 1800s competitive weight training originated. The first modern Olympics in 1896 had two Olympic lifts. The one- and two-hand lifts were used until the 1920s. In the 1920s weight classes were introduced and medals were given to the top three spots. Also in the 20s the lifts were developed into more of what we see in the Olympics today.

Eventually the lifts were broken down into three basic lifts using two hands: the snatch, the clean and jerk, and the press. The press was eventually discontinued and today we have the snatch and the clean and jerk. In both lifts a body position called the "full squat" is used to get the weight up. In the snatch the weight is "cleaned" from the floor and quickly dropped into a full squat position with the weight finishing over the head. The clean and jerk incorporated a power clean dropping into a full front squat and the weight is jerked overhead with a split lunge. The two lifts not only incorporate strength and power but speed and athletic ability as well.

## The Snatch

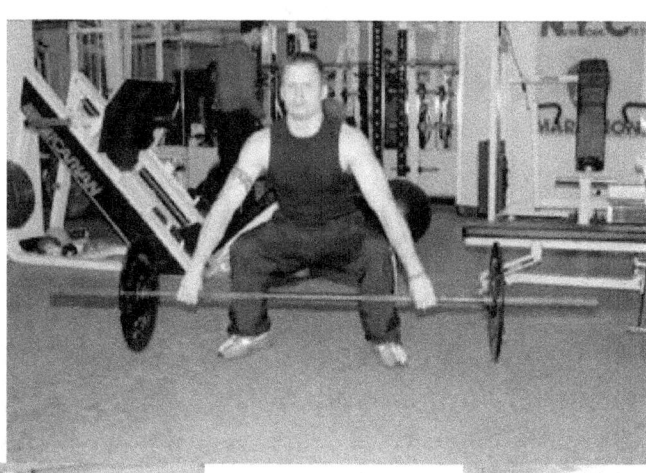

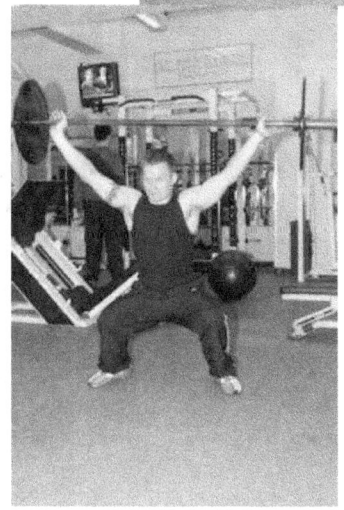

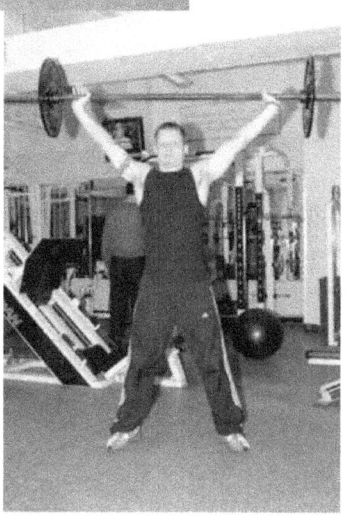

## Clean and Jerk

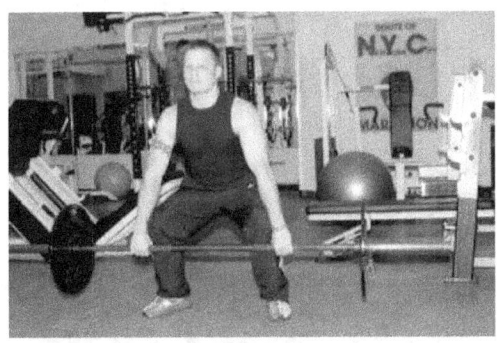

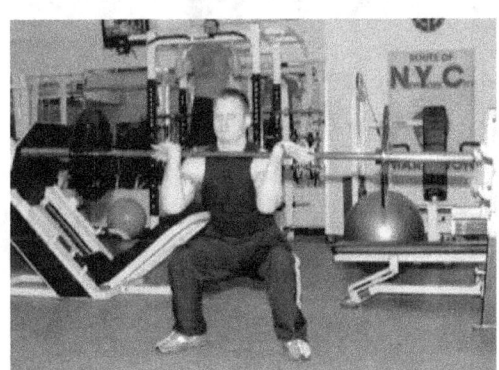

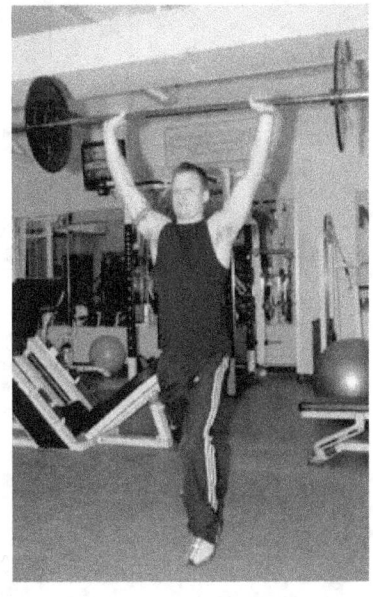

*Power Lifting Becomes Popular*

As more and more athletes became interested in Olympic lifting another sport, power lifting, became popular. Power lifting incorporated three major lifts.  These are the squat, dead lift, and bench press.

With the squat the bar is placed on the back and the competitor has to squat down to a parallel position and come up.

## Squat

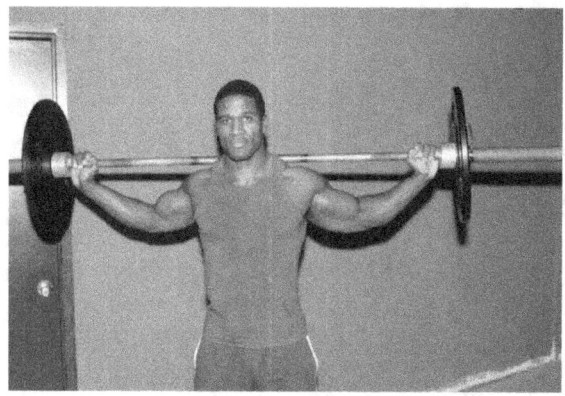

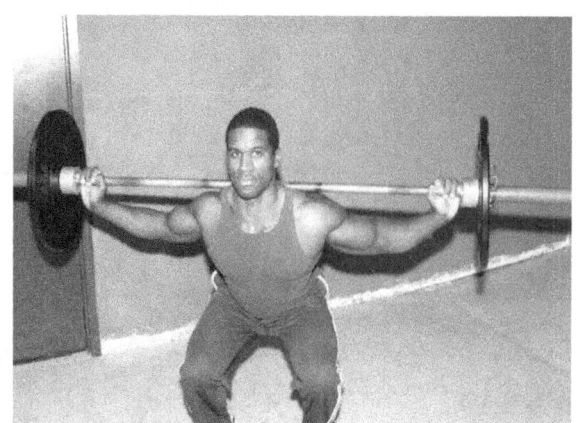

The deadlift is taken from the floor and the lifter has to pull the bar to a standing position with the arms hanging at the sides in a straight position.

## Dead Lift

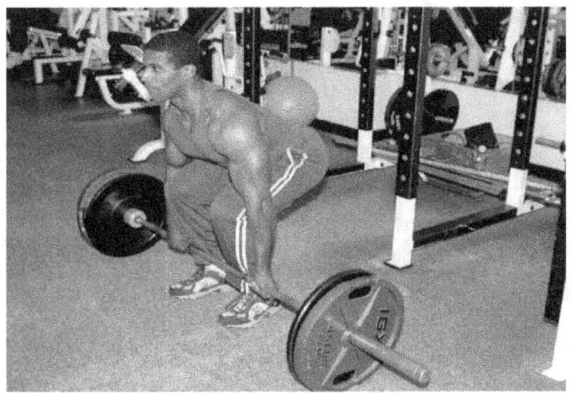

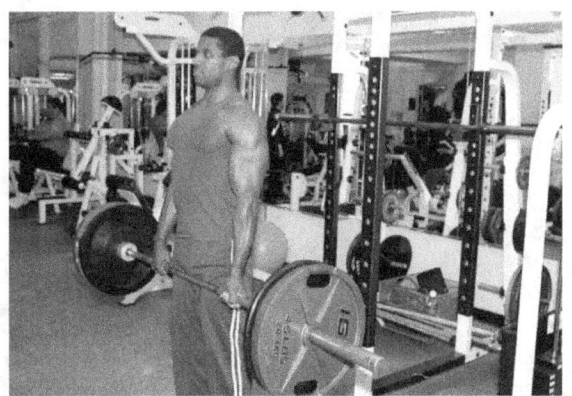

The bench press is a lift in which the lifter is lying on a flat bench and the weight is taken off the rack, held straight, and brought down to the middle part of the chest. The weight is held there for a split second until the lifter hears a clap and presses straight up. These three power lifts are pure power moves and don't take the athletic ability or speed the Olympic lifts take.

## Bench Press

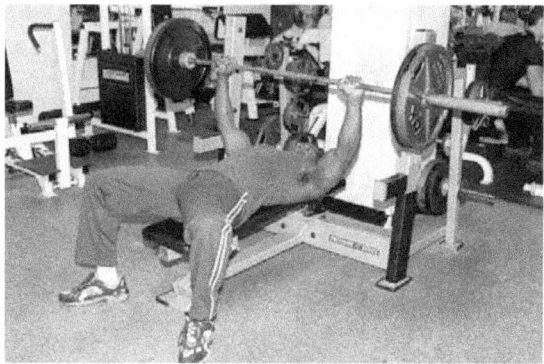

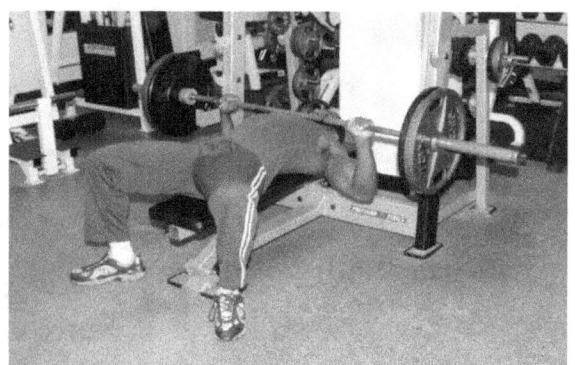

These three power lifts are incorporated in one form or another into most strength training routines today. The squat can be done in many different forms, the front squat with a barbell, back squat, the plie squat, squats with dumbbells, the one-legged squat, and many different forms of lunges.

The Bench Press can be done with dumbbells or barbells, or on the flat bench, incline bench, or decline bench.

From the combination of the Olympic lifts and power lifts hundreds of different exercises have been developed over the years.

## The Body Building Phenomenon

Body building competitions came about when barbell lifting became more popular.  Body building had been a very small sport in the 1940s and 50s.  There were few gyms where you could work out and only a handful of men lifted weights, usually in their own garages or at the YMCA. For a woman to lift weights was unheard of because weights – it was thought – would give them big muscles! No research had ever been done on strength training. It was assumed that lifting weights made you muscle-bound or very tight. Athletes who competed in sports such as boxing, basketball, and football would never lift weights because they thought it would reduce their agility and speed.

## Steve Reeves Begins To Change The View Of Body Building

There were a few people who actually began to change the consciousness of people about the potential of weight training. The first was a handsome young bodybuilder named – Steve Reeves.

Steve won the Mr. America title and Mr. Universe title in the late 40s and early 50s. He had become interested in bodybuilding at an early age when most people didn't know much about the sport. He had the kind of physique that men wanted and a look that women liked. His photographs were the inspiration of many aspiring bodybuilders and lifting weights began to gain in popularity. I remember seeing his pictures when I was a young boy. They certainly inspired me to start exercising at an early age.

In the 50s Steve became a star in the movies "Hercules" and "Hercules Unchained", changing the perception of bodybuilding forever. His pictures were seen in the first muscle magazines on the market. Reeves' natural body was developed before the use of steroids and his physique did not have the bulky look that so many of today's body builders develop. He went on to make many more movies in the 60s.

When he retired he began to write books about fitness and the workouts he did to develop his streamlined body. Today his picture can still be seen in many muscle and fitness magazines. Steve Reeves is known for his classic physique and is truly one of the greats who inspired millions in the fitness field.

*Can I Get The Key To The Weight Room?*

In the 70s before the fitness revolution started, the only gyms were in the major cities in the U.S. I can remember coming home from college and the only place to lift weights was the YMCA. The Y had a weight room that was about the size of a large bedroom. You had to go to the front desk to get the key to open it because hardly anyone used it! After my workout I would return the key to the front desk and I was probably the only person that used the room the whole day.

Since I was on the track team I also had to run and stay in shape for the sprints. Since the track had snow on it in upstate New York, I would find a clean patch of road to do my sprints. More than once the police would stop me and ask what I was running from! A few years later, and thanks to a handful of pioneers, things changed radically.

## Joe Weider's *Musclebuilder* Magazine

One of the pioneers was a man named Joe Weider. Joe started a magazine called "*Musclebuilder*" that was basically for men interested in bodybuilding. Joe Weider eventually started a bodybuilding organization called the IFBB, the "International Federation of Body Building". Another pioneer fitness guru, Bob Hoffman, started a competitive magazine called "*Strength and Health*". His magazine was geared toward Olympic lifters and athletes. Eventually Joe Weider became the more popular of the two and soon brought over a young body builder from Austria named – Arnold Schwarzenager. Joe used Arnold in his magazine to demonstrate bodybuilding routines and eventually this little-known Austrian began winning most major bodybuilding competitions from Mr. America to Mr. Universe.

## Arnold Schwarzenager Dominates Body Building

Arnold eventually won the IFBB professional Mr. Olympia contest in the 70s, and dominated the show by winning it seven straight times. He beat some of the sport's great bodybuilders – guys who had been seen on the cover of bodybuilding magazines. Arnold won against Frank Zane who eventually won again after Arnold retired. To this day at 66 years old Frank is still in competitive shape. Franco Columbo, who competed on TV in "The world's strongest man" contest, was beaten out by the young Austrian. Sergio Olivia, Mike Katz, and Lou Ferrigno – who became the Hulk on TV – were all unable to win against Arnold.

Arnold's movie career actually began with a documentary called "Pumping Iron".   Filmed in the 70s, it showed Arnold and Lou Ferrigno training and competing in the Mr. Olympia contest held in South Africa that year. The movie was very popular and inspired millions to take up the sport of fitness and bodybuilding.  Arnold's second movie was called "Stay Hungry" and starred Sally Fields and Jeff Bridges. Arnold played the part of a bodybuilder who worked out in the gym in a batman costume and got into a relationship with Sally

Fields. The movie would probably be even more popular today than it was back in the early 70s. Arnold retired from bodybuilding only to land the role as Conan in the movie "Conan the Barbarian".

In the second Conan movie, "Conan the Destroyer", Arnold needed to have a better physique so he began training hard again. Arnold looked so good that he came out of retirement and won the Mr. Olympia title one more time, with the competition being the strongest that he ever went up against. These men were legends in their sport:  Mike Menzner, Boyer Coe, Frank Zane, Dennis Tinarino, all of them beaten by Arnold.

Today Arnold can still be seen in bodybuilding magazines along with the legends he once defeated. The rest is history – the history of an action movie superstar!  Arnold was an inspiration to millions of people to start working out and donated his time to promote physical fitness among young people. The discipline required to build his body has served him well in public office as the governor of California.  He is truly one of the greats in the history of body building and in promoting health and physical fitness.

## Muscle Beach and Gold's Gyms

The sport of bodybuilding continued to grow as more and more men entered competitions.  Gyms began to open up throughout the US, especially in California.  Muscle Beach in Venice, California became well known and the Gold's Gym chains began to open up throughout the country.

## Jack LaLanne – Fitness Guru

Another pioneer in helping to develop the health and fitness field is a man named Jack LaLanne. He started weight training at an early age and developed a great body. In the early 60s he had his own exercise program for women on TV and even had nutrition tips on the show. Through the years he was well known for his physical feats of strength and endurance. One such feat was to swim handcuffed from Alcatraz Island towing a row boat with an enormous amount of weight in it!

Jack LaLanne was indeed a fitness guru and as he got older he continued to test himself with his amazing feats. Eventually he opened a chain of health and fitness clubs and even today he can be seen on TV advertising a new health product. He continues to work out with intensity daily, at the age of 93. The name Jack LaLanne is well known in the fitness industry and he had a huge influence in helping to develop the health and fitness field.

## Arthur Jones' Nautilus Gyms

During this same time Arthur Jones developed a line of exercise equipment known as "Nautilus". Back in the early 80s I was opening a Nautilus Fitness Center in Alexandria, Virginia and traveled to Jones' home in Deland Florida for a seminar and to purchase some Nautilus equipment for my gym. His motto was "younger women, bigger crocodiles, and faster airplanes"! Jones, who was 62 at the time, had an 18-year-old girlfriend and I can remember seeing a huge crocodile fenced in his yard!

At that time his one-set method of training was controversial to most bodybuilders. At a time when gyms were opening around the country Jones had developed a system in which he used one set on each machine to failure. Working "to failure" means to perform repetitions until you are physically unable to do more. The workout took no more than thirty minutes. His system was controversial in that other fitness experts insisted that free weights were better than any machine. My final conclusion was that Jones' system was good but by incorporating free weights with it you got more of a complete workout. Free weights require balance and flexibility that machines don't. Arthur Jones marketed his Nautilus machines and soon Nautilus Fitness Centers sprouted up all across the country.

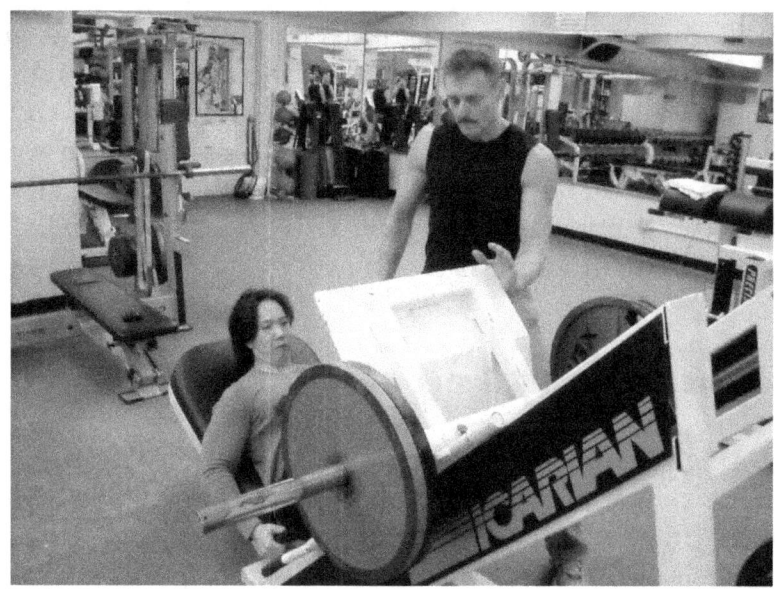

*Machines plus free weights provide the best workout.*

## Going For The Burn In The 80s

In the 1980s weight training and exercise became popular not just with the average man who wanted to develop his body, but with women and athletes as well. Gyms were thriving and many other fitness and bodybuilding magazines began to arise. Soon other countries began to follow the U.S. in the fitness revolution and today you can usually find a place to work out in almost any country in the world. Scientific studies began to support strength training for people of different ages. Fitness videos became the rage, people were going "for the burn", and everyone wanted to look good.

## Millions of Baby Boomers Want To Stay "Forever Young"

Today it's not just about looking good but about feeling good and staying healthy as well. Gyms have become "fitness centers" with saunas, racquetball courts, and health food cafes. As one of the largest age cohorts in history – the baby boomers – enter their 50s and 60s, health and fitness have become mainstream. We want to look better, eat better, and feel better – longer. Science tells us how to accomplish this – through a combination of cardio exercise and strength training. This is exactly what we have done in the **Younger Body Now** routines we've developed.   Through my years of experience as a personal trainer, I have seen my older clients begin to feel better and younger and my younger clients improve their fitness levels. Even clients who have not started training until their 50s have continued to improve their fitness levels into their late 60s.

*Older clients feel younger.  Younger clients improve fitness levels.*

I have also had clients with osteoporosis gain bone density in one year. Clients with mobility problems are more active than ever before. My clients feel better and their quality of life improves. Instead of slowing down they're gearing up for the rest of their lives. Building on over 100 years of the history of weight training, along with the latest research on the science of aging, the routines we've developed will get you *off the couch and back in the game*.

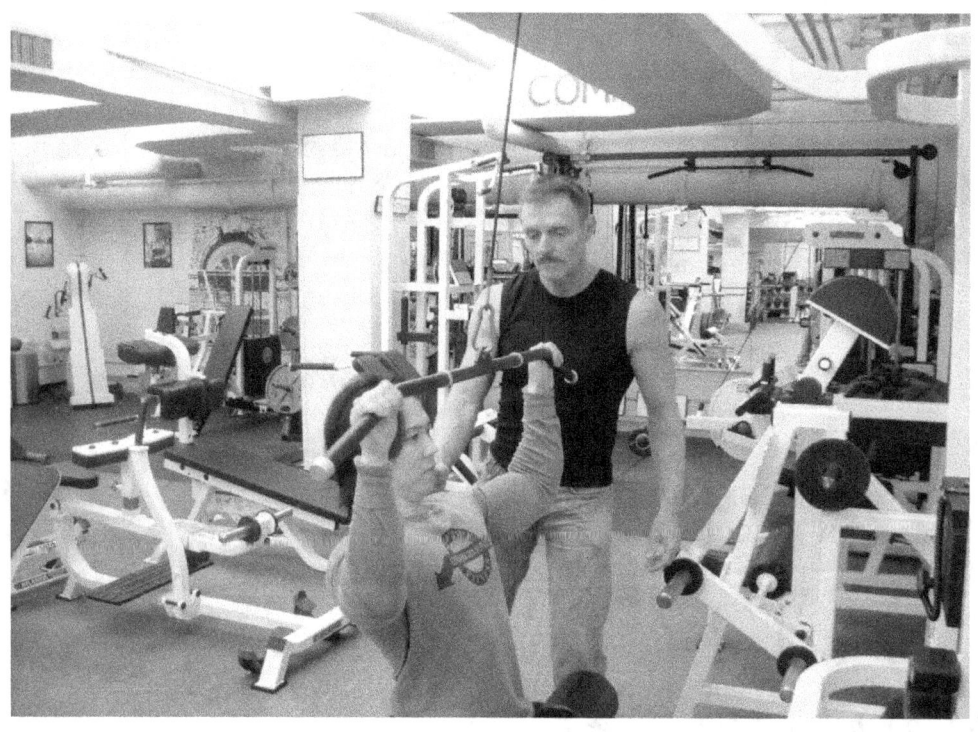

# 3

## The Research Says It All

So how strong is the science behind the **Younger Body Now** concepts? Very strong.

Recently many Americans were surprised to learn from research that fit people who were still overweight tend to outlive their slimmer peers who are less fit.[1]   Steven Blair, professor at the University of South Carolina Arnold School of Public Health, noted "Older individuals need to be concerned about their fitness level.  There is perhaps too much focus on body weight, and fitness is only an afterthought".

When I was competing in mountain bike racing I had a friend named Doug who used to train with me a couple times a week. Doug was no great athlete and he was about 50 pounds overweight but had drive and desire and never gave up at anything. We would ride in the woods on some pretty hard and hairy trails but he always managed to finish the workout no matter what the challenge was. There was a steep three-mile climb called Devil's Kitchen that we would ride once a week. It was one of those climbs that got steeper and steeper as you got closer to the top, and was certainly a mental and physical challenge to finish the climb. Well, Doug would always amaze me. No matter how long it took he would always make that climb.

One weekend I brought a couple of fit-looking trainers from New York City to do some mountain biking with us. We went to some easy trails in the woods because I didn't want to take them anywhere they might get hurt. The pace was fairly slow and it was a fun ride and not a day to get a hard workout in. At one point we came to a pretty steep hill about a half mile long. We all started out together and eventually Doug made it to the top, leaving the two fit-looking trainers walking their bikes up the hill. When they got to the top they were totally shocked that this overweight person could crush them on a hill. They asked me how it was possible that Doug could ride all the way to the top and they couldn't. I replied "he may look fat but he's the one who's fit." My two friends learned an important lesson that day. Just because you look fit doesn't necessarily mean you really are.

## Physical Activity Impacts Health

The Centers for Disease Control and Prevention, National Center for Chronic Disease Prevention and Health Promotion notes how physical activity impacts health.[2] They note regular physical activity impacts health in the following ways:

- Reduces risk of premature death
- Reduces risk of dying prematurely from heart disease
- Reduces likelihood of developing diabetes
- Lessons risk of developing high blood pressure
- Reduces risk of colon cancer
- Improves weight control
- Helps maintain health bones, muscles, and joints
- Helps older adults build strength and mobility
- Promotes psychological wellbeing

A growing body of research supports strength training in particular as a critical part of a total fitness program. The July/August 2002 issue of American Fitness[3] notes that muscle strength is an essential component of optimal health, function, well-being, and quality of life. They note that as we age we tend to lose as much as 30 percent or more of our muscular strength as well as muscle mass. They confirm that this loss can be reversed through strength training. They go on to explain other key outcomes of strength training:

- Improved body composition
- Better glucose metabolism
- Better functional ability for daily activities
- Better body image and higher self esteem
- Higher metabolism
- Increased energy
- Stronger bones
- Less back pain
- Reduced stress and better sleep
- Overall improved quality of life

They note that the American College of Sports Medicine provided specific guidelines in 1998 for muscle strength and endurance training. These included exercising all major muscle groups two to three days per week using one set of 8 – 12 repetitions for healthy adults. Older adults were suggested to use 10 –15 repetitions.

These guidelines were updated in 2002, and now emphasize the importance of more individualized training programs working with trained exercise specialists. Our workout plan fulfills these research-based recommendations. The guidelines now refer to "resistance training" which provides continuous improvement on a specific area such as muscle strength, power, etc. They note that resistance training is proven to enhance speed, coordination, balance, flexibility, and overall motor performance. The ACSM also notes that progress over the long term requires variety in volume and intensity – key components of our program as well.

## Squats – A Key Component Of Your Younger Body Now Workout

Gains in muscle strength are noted to come through multiple-joint exercises such as squats – a key component of our client's personal training. Squats work knee and hip joints and target the quadriceps, hamstrings, and gluteal muscles. Using free weights are also noted to improve core stabilizer muscles to help maintain body posture and balance. These multi-joint exercises also improve muscle power with shorter, more intense workouts.

The ACSM guidelines also say that healthy older adults should use progressive resistance training. The guidelines again emphasize the importance of working with qualified trainers. **Our system is like having your own personal trainer!**

One of the best-known exercise scientists in the world today, Dr. William Kraemer of the University of Connecticut, is also a noted proponent of weight training.[4] Dr. Kraemer developed and has edited the Journal of Strength and Conditioning Research for over 20 years and is well known for putting his research into practice.  He has studied the effects of resistance training on bone, variation in growth hormones, muscle, the body's endocrine and immune systems, the problems of over-training, and the impact of resistance training on women and older adults.  He has conducted research and provided consulting for the International Olympic Committee, NASA, and the Department of Defense.

Dr. Kraemer's book, "Designing Resistance Training Programs", written with another leading expert, Steven J. Fleck, again demonstrates the scientific knowledge behind personalized training programs. In Men's Fitness, October 2003[5], Kraemer notes squats (a key component of our program)  as the single best exercise for legs. He comments that squats provide the compound movement that stimulates all the major leg muscles. He defines squats as one of the pillars of strength-fitness exercise, and suggests working the legs from a variety of angles and postures to stimulate as many muscle fibers as possible.

## Strength Training Benefits Our Most Senior Citizens

There is also ongoing research on the need for exercise and strength training for older adults. Dr. Maria Fiatarone Singh, professor of Medicine and Sports Science at the University of Sydney in Australia, writes that the best medicine for old age is exercise![6] Writing for the Alliance for Aging Research Fall 2001 she reports a study of strength training on frail adults in their 80s and 90s in Boston. Nearly all the participants had arthritis and heart disease and were on multiple medications. Most used walkers and had experienced falls. Within ten weeks of beginning a strength-training program, the researchers saw across the board improvements. Participants got stronger, could walk faster and climb stairs more easily, and became more sociable. No such improvements were apparent in the control group.

Dr. Singh advocates strength and balance training for anyone with difficulty walking, who falls, or who is susceptible to fractures. She also states that chronic, age-related medical conditions almost always indicate a need for exercise. Her work suggests that depression is well treated with exercise, with weight lifting and aerobic exercise working equally well. She says strength training shows improvements in just a few weeks, and reports that older adults tend to stay with strength training even when they drop out of aerobic work such as cycling or walking.

## Health Problems Are A Reason For Exercise, Not An Excuse To Avoid It!

Dr. Singh reiterates what we say at **Younger Body Now** – It's never too late to start! She recommends seeing health problems as a reason *FOR* exercise not a barrier to it, and encourages everyone to look for opportunities to exercise rather than reasons to avoid it.

As we have seen above, the 1998 position of the American College of Sports Medicine[7] on exercise for older adults supports the notion that endurance and strength training can help maintain and improve various aspects of cardiovascular functioning, cardiac output, and reduce risk factors associated with diseases such as heart disease and diabetes. It is also known to improve overall health status and increase life expectancy. Strength training in particular helps offset muscle mass loss as well as bone loss. It improves posture, reduces the risk of falling, and increases flexibility and range of motion.

These recommendations have recently been updated and differentiated for older adults as well. In cooperation with the American Heart Association in August, 2007[8] the ACSM provided in-depth recommendations for physical activity and public health in older adults. They specifically recommend activities that maintain or increase flexibility and balance exercises. They note that a fitness program for older adults should emphasize moderate intensity aerobic activity, muscle-strengthening activity, and reduce sedentary behavior.

## Increased Activity Now Can Reduce Health Costs Later

They go on to predict that increasing levels of activity among older adults could reduce their medical expenditures within a year. They recommend the following muscle-strengthening activities – along with aerobic exercise – for improvement of specific chronic illnesses:

**All healthy adults:**  at least two days/week of 8-10 exercises involving all major muscle groups.

**Older adults:**  at least two days/week of 8-10 exercises involving all major muscle groups with increasing repetitions

**For bone health and osteoporosis:**  two-three days/week of a progressive program of weight training that uses all muscle groups of sufficient intensity; include balance in the overall training program

**For cardiovascular disease:**  two to three days/week of 8-10 exercises involving all major muscle groups

**For hypertension:**  two – three days/week including resistance training of 8-10 exercises involving all major muscle groups

**For type-2 diabetes:** three days/week for all major muscle groups

**For high cholesterol:** muscle strengthening and flexibility regarded as beneficial

**For stroke:** two – three days/week of 8-10 exercises for all major muscle groups with two – three days/week of flexibility training

**For osteoarthritis:** two – three days/week of isotonic resistance exercises involving all major muscle groups, and three-five days/week of flexibility

The **Younger Body Now** regimen is successful because it follows not only my own years of experience, but my son's as well, and the scientifically-based recommendations of the leading health organizations in America today. As the American Heart Association notes, regular physical activity that include aerobics and strength training is essential for healthy aging. It reduces the risk of chronic disease, premature mortality, and disability. It's the way to a **Younger Body – Now**!

As other studies have pointed out, the Heart Association confirms the need for a "plan" for obtaining the required activity levels and strength training needs. **Younger Body Now** provides just such a plan. They point out that historically, people maintained their strength through routine physical activity such as farming and manufacturing. Today we have become much more sedentary. The Association recommends a planned program of strength training, flexibility, and balance as essential for healthy aging in today's more knowledge-based society.

More and more research is being compiled, and recommendations being made, regarding the health and fitness needs of older adults. The Center for Disease Control is promoting an initiative to ensure that community planners are on board with the need to facilitate a more active lifestyle for community members.[9] They report the following facts:

- The loss of strength and stamina with aging is caused in part by reduced physical activity
- Inactivity increases with age; 1/3 of all adults 75 or older engage in no physical activity
- Older adults benefit from regular physical activity
- In addition to aerobics, older adults benefit from strength training
- Such training can help control joint swelling and the pain associated with arthritis
- Improvements are noted in bone health, muscles, and joints
- Organized physical activities should include strength training and flexibility components.

*Only 5.6% Of Adults Meet National Objectives For Physical Activity and Strength Training*

The CDC also says that strength training helps adults improve their overall health and fitness as well as improving insulin sensitivity and glucose metabolism. In fact a national health objective for 2010 is to increase to 30% the proportion of adults who perform physical activities that maintain muscular strength and endurance two or more days per week [10.] They say that most older adults, even those who are otherwise active, are missing opportunities to improve their overall health and fitness through regular strength training. Only 5.6% of Americans meet national objectives for both physical activity and strength training. **The Younger Body Now program is designed to help you reach the national goal.**

A January 31, 2008, New York Times article shows even more support[11]. In "Staying a Step Ahead of Aging" Dr. Vonda Wright, a professor of orthopedics at the University of Pittsburgh and a 40-year-old runner, studied people who kept training as they got older or began competing in middle age to find when their performance started to decline. Surprisingly, the investigators found that even if you start training later in life, you can stave off more of the deterioration than you thought through exercise. One man in the study took up running at 62 and ran his first marathon, a year later, in 3 hours 25 minutes. The article does indicate you have to know how to train, what exercises to do, and you have to keep it up!

"Train hard and train often," said Hirofumi Tanaka, a 41-year-old soccer player and exercise physiologist at the University of Texas[12]. This means regular interval training in which you go full out, ease up, then go full out again to increase your oxygen consumption. According to Dr. Tanaka you have to make training "as intense as you can".

*Train hard and train often!*

Steve Hawkins, an exercise physiologist at the University of Southern California, says working out hard is more important that working out often[13]. "High performance is really determined more by intensity than volume," he notes. "Sometimes, when you're older, something has to give. You can't have both so you have to cut back on the volume.

Older athletes can have spectacular performances, Dr. Tanaka notes in the Times article. The world's best marathon time for men 70 or older, 2:54:05, was set by a 74-year-old. That's better than the winning marathon time at the first modern Olympics, the 1896 Games in Athens!

"I'm a CFO for a big corporation and I used to work out an hour with another trainer. Since I started Art's 30-minute workout I have gotten better results and I look and feel great. It's better than anything I've ever tried."

...Pat Spille, 62

*4*

## The Role of Healthy Eating In Getting A Younger Body Now

### Diet To Lose Weight Or Eat Healthy To Live Well?

First I want to clarify the difference between a weight-loss diet and eating in a healthy manner.  Most people who want to lose weight want to do it very quickly so they choose a diet or system that they have read about or seen advertised on TV.  The list of famous diets is endless but in reality most diets will work if you stick with them.  Still let's face it, who wants to be on a diet for the rest of their life?  Any time we cut our calories down to a minimum and we burn more calories than we take in, we are going to lose weight.  This is probably a good thing because we all know that the thinner we are the healthier we are, right?  Well that's not necessarily true.  Let me explain why.

If you take a person that weighs 180 pounds and their body fat is 30%, then they go on a diet and lose 30 pounds, what would their body fat be?  The answer is 30%!  What they have lost is an equal amount of fat and muscle and in reality what you have is a smaller, but still "fat" person!  So what's the answer?  What we really want to do is change our body fat composition, and by doing so we want to burn fat and increase muscle at the same time.  We lose fat and gain muscle by eating correctly and by being on a good exercise program.

## Types Of Dieters

Through the years I have trained many people who wanted to lose weight or lose body fat and gain muscle.  Basically I have dealt with four types of people and diets:

- Body builders who wanted to get lean before a show and get down to a very low percentage of body fat,
- People who were overweight and wanted to lose weight to look better,
- Athletes who wanted to improve their performance, and
- People who wanted to eat healthy to combat the effects of disease such as heart disease, cancer, diabetes, etc.

I'm going to discuss all four types together because I feel it is important to understand every aspect of dieting. Anyone can put these principles into their own life – whatever your motivation for changing your eating habits.

First of all I want to say that the biggest mistake most people make when they are dieting is that they don't eat enough.  They think that if they skip meals and starve themselves the pounds will drop off.  Yes, you will lose weight at first, but when your body takes in let's say, 800 calories a day, it will have a tendency to hold on to more fat and burn muscle for energy instead – the opposite of what you want to accomplish.  Of course there are a few ways to counteract this, one being to try and build muscle while you are dieting through weight training.

When I was training my clients for a bodybuilding show and they had eight weeks before the show, I would encourage them to cut out all white sugar and white flour.  I would also encourage them to cut down their consumption of fat.  In addition I would tell them to eat six small meals per day as this would increase their metabolism so they would actually burn fat.

The secret here is also about what you are actually eating!  When I trained someone for a body building show, or when I was training for one myself, I made sure there were enough calories and nutrition to maintain a high level of training.  The food was always healthy of course. When I wanted to lose body fat for a show I always consumed more frequent but smaller meals consisting of the right kinds of food.  It is always easier to cut out the wrong foods but eat more of the good foods when you are dieting.  So a body builder trying to lose body fat and maintain muscle mass has to do basically the same thing as anyone who just wants to lose weight and look good, male or female.

*Eating six times a day to lose weight?  Sounds good!*

Setting up a nutritional program for athletes was a bit different, especially for runners.  Cutting out the bad food was basically the same but runners need to consume more clean, complex, carbohydrates.  By that I mean brown rice instead of white rice, 7-grain or stone ground whole wheat bread instead of white bread, and no white sugar.  Of course this would eliminate a wide variety of foods because most processed foods contain sugar.  Still this leaves us with a wide variety of healthy and delicious foods to choose from.  I will share the foods I eat as part of my own fitness program but before that I want to focus on the important mental outlook necessary for weight loss.

## Focusing On Weight Loss Is A Recipe For Failure

First of all when potential clients come to see me I ask them what their goals are.  If they tell me they want to get fitter, healthier, stronger, and look better, I will take them on as a client since I know I can help them be successful with those goals.  If they say they want to lose weight as their main goal I send them to someone else.  I believe people who just want to lose weight without looking at overall health and fitness are setting themselves up for failure.  Losing weight and being healthy go hand in hand.   Both require a lifestyle change.  By that I mean getting on a daily exercise routine and changing your eating habits.  Getting healthier has to become part of your daily life and you gradually have to change the way you think.

*People who just want to lose weight are setting themselves up for failure.*

## Weight Loss Success – And Failure

When I was in the gym business I had a 36-year-old woman who came to me and said she had a dream of being in a bodybuilding show.  She weighed 228 pounds and had to lose at least 100 pounds to do so.  I told her what she had to do which was to totally change the way she ate and work out with weights and cardio six times per week.  I was a little bit skeptical because from experience I know how hard it is to completely change your body.  It would take daily supervision and tremendous will power.

Some of us watch the show on TV called the "Biggest Loser" where people lose over 100 pounds in a fairly short amount of time.  Let me tell you that these people are in an atmosphere where they live, eat, and breathe exercise with trained professionals at their side all day.  This isn't a typical situation for most people because it's not like real life.

What happened to my 36-year-old client you're asking?   I worked out my client six times per week and told her about the right foods to eat and what to avoid. If she was going out with her family on a Friday night she knew she needed to think about just how many pieces of pizza she could have!  She began losing weight – 10, 20, 30 pounds.  Her appearance began to change and she felt more attractive as she lost the weight. Unfortunately, her husband who was overweight himself, became insecure in their relationship.

My client did lose the 100 pounds but it took almost a year.  We prepared her for the bodybuilding show and she got last place in her class.  Still she looked and felt great and she certainly was considered competitive by the judges.  No one questioned if she deserved to be there.  She had come a long way in a year and she was happy at the time with the results she attained.  She looked like a totally different person.

Although she appeared very attractive and outwardly confident, the person inside was still the same.  She told me that when she looked in the mirror she still saw the same overweight woman she used to be. Psychologically she wasn't ready for the change and perhaps her motives weren't the right ones.  She had achieved her goal of getting in shape for a bodybuilding show – she eventually did another show with the same outcome – but the weight eventually came back.  I learned a lesson as a trainer from that experience. If you put fitness and health first, all else will follow.  If you don't, a short-term success can become a long-term failure.  Be patient with yourself and enjoy the results for the rest of your life.

When a client comes to me now and tells me their only goal is to lose weight, I know they are setting themselves up for failure.  Their goals should be to become fit and healthy.  If they work at that goal they will succeed.

*You will love getting stronger and fitter.  Looking good is icing on the cake!*

When my clients go to the gym they love the experience of getting stronger and fitter and having more energy and a better quality of life. When their appearance changes too, it's icing on the cake! If you focus on feeling younger, feeling better, and being able to do the things you did 5, 10, or 20 year ago, you will succeed.

"Since I have been doing the short intense 30-minute workout, my body fat has gone down 7% and I've dropped two dress sizes. I'm in the best shape of my life."

Amanda Rosen, 40

*5*

## So What Do You Eat For A Younger Body Now?

### A Healthy Eating Plan

Now that we've got our mind in the right place, let's talk a little bit about the foods we can eat or should eat to be healthy. We know that eating four to six times per day is ideal and drinking water is a necessity. The reader should consult his or her own physician before starting any diet or exercise program. There are many diet and nutrition resources available as well. My goal here is to share what I have found works well for my clients – I know it works for me.

When I first started training in Manhattan, my clients wanted a diet to lose weight. Even though I was against the idea, I devised a diet that everyone could do without starving themselves. The plan was a low carb diet with moderate fat intake with no more than 50 to 75 grams of carbs per day. It would be three days on, one day off, or five days on and two days off. The "off" day did not mean you could eat everything in sight! The off days mean to be responsible, not consume more than 200 grams of carbs per day, and of course eat the right foods. The diet is simple and is drawn from today's typical recommendations for healthy eating:

- All the steamed fresh vegetables and salad you wanted,
- three-four protein servings per day from meat, fish, chicken, turkey, lean pork, tuna, veal, or whatever lean fresh meat you wanted, no deli meat,
- two fruits per day, and
- one complex carb such as two slices of 7-grain or sprouted organic bread, one yam, oatmeal, organic cereal, or six ounces of brown rice.

I avoid pasta on diet days. The fruit and complex carbs would come out to be between 75 to 100 grams of carbs per day. One yogurt could be substituted for a fruit. Four ounces of cheese could be used in place of a protein. Also I try not to eat any complex carbs after 5 pm. A protein, fruit, yogurt, cheese, or vegetables are OK.

The beverages I consume include carrot juice, water, coffee, or tea and small amounts of skim milk. Clients often ask about diet drinks. They do seem to help the craving for sugar and I have to admit I've used them myself before a bodybuilding show.

A sample diet plan might be as follows:

**Sample 1**

**Breakfast:** an omelet of two eggs (2 whites and 1 yolk), bowl of oatmeal or organic cereal, one piece of fruit

**Snack:** one piece of fruit or a yogurt

**Lunch:** tuna salad or green salad with chicken breast

Whey protein shake

**Dinner:** salad, steamed vegetables, 6 ounces of protein, fish, chicken, and meat in that order

**Snack:** 4 ounces cheese

## Sample 2

**Breakfast:** 3-egg omelet with cheese (3 whites and 1 yolk), 1 piece fruit

**Snack:** protein shake (whey protein), skim milk or water

**Lunch:** tuna sandwich or any meat on organic 7-grain bread with lettuce and tomato

**Snack:** fruit

**Dinner:** salad, steamed vegetables and 6 ounces protein

**Snack:** 4 ounces cheese

Again this diet is either the three days on one day off or five days on two days off. There are no fried foods, white sugar, or white products on the diet!

Remember that diets are a short term fix. I only recommend dieting if a person has to lose weight for some special event – like a 25th high school reunion - where they just have to look good!

If you burn more calories than you consume, no matter what the diet is you will lose weight. Be active and if you are just starting out, do what you can. Walk every day, twice a day, three times a day! If you just can't do that much, do what you can and gradually increase it. Make exercise a daily part of your routine. Do some form of exercise every day. If you feel tired at the end of the day when you come home from work, go for a walk, do your workout, or go to the gym! Many times my clients would say they almost cancelled that day but they forced themselves to come in. Every single person who came in to work out was glad they did and felt wide awake and energized when they left. I've never had a case where someone felt worse after one of my workouts!

## What's The Case For Supplements To Feel Younger Now?

## Supplementing A Healthy Diet

Today we read and hear about all the different supplements that we should be taking.   There are many different health and fitness magazines and most of them advocate that we should take certain supplements.   In the last 25 years I have studied the supplement industry and I myself and many of my clients have used most of the supplements out there.   Of course everyone should check with their doctor to determine their need for supplements and whether supplements may interfere with any medication they are taking.

Instead of going over every single vitamin, mineral, herb, and supplement on the market, let's keep it simple and just list those that seem to be the most important. These include the ones I and my clients and athletes have had the most success with.   Again there is a wealth of information on supplements available for further research by the reader.

Considering vitamins first, the question we ask ourselves is do we get enough vitamins from our foods?  Some people tell me they eat a well-balanced diet so they must be getting all the vitamins they need.  Well if everyone was eating a well-balanced diet there would be less problems with diseases such as cancer, heart disease, or diabetes. Can't I just eat a balanced diet and be done with it?  No, because the soil has become so depleted through the years that a lot of our foods aren't as healthy as they used to be.   Our animals are fed hormones, our plants have harmful sprays, and the list goes on.   Everywhere we look we hear that something else we are eating causes cancer.  So what do we do, eat all organic foods?  I can tell you that eating all organic is not easy and it certainly isn't cheap.  Most of us aren't going to do it on a regular basis – including me.

## My Top Five

Instead of listing all the different supplements I take, and since this isn't a nutrition book, I'm going to list the top five supplements that many nutritionists and doctors recommend. These are also the ones I have had most success with:

1. **Probiotics** – This is the good bacteria in our intestines. Probiotics are essential for the absorption of nutrients and help get rid of the bad bacteria. This good bacteria helps in our digestive system and is very healthy for our immune system. Probiotics bring back a proper balance of good and bad bacteria in our intestinal tract.

2. **Omega 3 – 6 – 9** – The Omegas come from fish and plant sources and provide the essential fatty acids that we need. Essential fatty acids are responsible for healthy skin, hair, joint flexibility, and normal fat metabolism. There have been many studies done on the benefits of fish oil in our body. Some of the health benefits are a stronger heart, healthier arteries, freedom from inflammation, lower blood pressure, the prevention of colon cancer, and a reduction in the risk of stroke. We also get our omegas from flax seed oil. Flax seed oil is known for its beneficial effects on arthritis and the joints. I have found that when my athletic clients take omegas they seem to have an increase in energy and endurance

3. **Vitamin E** – (gamma E) There have been many studies done on the benefits of vitamin E. Vitamin E is a wonderful antioxidant that helps to neutralize free radical in our body. Free radicals can come from the air we breathe, chemicals in our food, or even too much stress. We know that free radicals cause damage and disease in our body. Vitamin E is also good for the heart and I feel that it definitely should be on anyone's top five list.

4. **Vitamin C** – Some people may disagree with me but I tend to support most of the things Dr. Linus Pauling wrote about vitamin C. It is good for the immune system and works well to keep our body

healthy and prevent disease.  Although I don't believe in the mega doses Dr. Pauling recommended, I think it is an important vitamin to take.  When I buy vitamin C I prefer to have bioflavonoids included in it.  I also prefer to take Ester C.

5. **CoQ10** – CoQ10 is produced in our body and is found in every cell, especially in the heart.  As we age our CoQ10 levels decline which eventually could weaken the heart.  CoQ10 is especially good for our cardiovascular health and helps prevent strokes, heart attacks, and high blood pressure.

## Worth More Research

Since this is not a nutrition book I won't go over all the supplements we could take.  I do think everyone should do their own research to learn more about some fabulous supplements that can benefit your health.  In addition to my top five, it is a good idea to take a good multi-vitamin. Below I list what I think are some other supplements to consider:

- **Whey protein:** a supplement I recommend for anyone that is working out is whey protein. Most athletes incorporate whey protein in their supplements because it has all the essential amino acids our body needs to build muscle.  Try and get a whey protein supplement that contains extra glutamine.  Glutamine helps prevent muscle breakdown before and after a workout and speeds up recovery.

- **B-Complex** : the stress supplement. B vitamins are good for the nervous system, skin, and muscles.

- **Magnesium**: Magnesium is an important mineral good for the bones, blood sugar level, blood pressure, and for cardio vascular disease.

- **Potassium:** a mineral that helps balance the electrolytes in your body and also helps regulate heart rate

- **NAC-Acetyl-L-Cysteine**: a supplement that is well worth looking into.  It is a precursor to glutathione which is good for the immune system.

- **Acetyl-L-Carnitine:**  good for brain function and heart health and may also help burn body fat

- **Zinc:** Zinc is a mineral that supports a healthy immune system and wound healing.

- **Saw Palmetto Berry Extract:** helps maintain a healthy prostate

- **Alpha Lipoic Acid:** a powerful antioxidant good for cardio-vascular health, brain function, helps the immune system and protects the liver

- **Beta 1, 3 Glucans**: known to treat autoimmune diseases and is well worth researching

- **Calcium:** essential for healthy bones and teeth

- **Glucosamine**: a natural compound found in healthy cartilage. Glucosamine may help to repair joint and damaged cartilage and is widely used for osteoarthritis.

- **Beta-Carotene:** a carotenoid that can be converted to vitamin A and is good for maintaining vision and proper function of the immune system

I highly recommend the following super foods as an addition to your diet:

- Wheat grass
- Spirulina
- Chlorella
- Barley grass
- Blue green algae

These super foods are high in chlorophyll and not only detoxify the body, but give us energy as well. Each of the super foods has its own life-giving properties and does much for your immune system to help keep your body healthy.

I like to keep my diet as natural as possible. I eat whole grains, fresh fruits and vegetables, plenty of fish – at least twice a week – organic eggs and poultry if possible, and less meat. This puts me on the road to optimum health. Shopping at the health food section in the supermarket or at a regular health food store allows me to buy the other food products that I need in everyday life. I recommend you do the same. It's also important to cook with olive oil as a healthy choice. Organic eggs are high in the Omegas and I believe that the yolk is good for you because it is a good fat. I eat fish that are rich in the Omega 3 fatty acids such as salmon, sardines, tuna, and trout. It is also a good idea to drink your fruit juices freshly squeezed and to drink raw vegetable juices as often as you can. I also try to eat a raw salad every day and steamed vegetables once or twice a day. A diet high in fiber is also very important and whole grains such as brown and wild rice, steel cut oats, and organic whole grain breads help to lower cholesterol. I prefer almond milk over regular milk and when I do drink milk I buy organic skim milk. We all have our favorite foods to eat and everyone's diet is going to be different but eating healthy is a major part of staying young and reversing the aging process.

So, keeping it healthy is definitely part of my program. By eating healthy foods and exercising every day you will eventually feel like a new person. Someone once asked me what was more important, exercising or eating right. I said that they both go hand in hand but if I had a choice I would exercise.

The reason for my choice is that weight training reverses the aging process by keeping your bones, joints, muscles, and tendons strong. A diet alone can't do that. Also doing cardio along with the weight training keeps your heart strong and healthy. Combine this with eating healthy and the sky's the limit!

"Before I started doing these workouts with Art I had to hold my husband's hand walking down the street because my balance was so bad. Now I can do anything with no problem; my strength, bone density, and balance are great. I also lost fifteen pounds and I just feel fantastic!"

... Ruth Riemer, 76

# 6

## Starting A New Life – You're Younger Already!

### Don't Start By Joining A Gym!

You may have been much more active when you were younger. Back *then* you felt good and had lots of energy. *Now* you've become a couch potato. What's *next*? You've never exercised that much before and your diet isn't that great either, so what do you do? Well joining a gym is probably not the right answer – at least not right now. Being in the gym business I know that too many people join a gym, use it for a couple of weeks, then never return. Also if we are out of hope and over 50 it is really easy to become intimidated.

What I suggest is to get into the habit of exercising for at least three months before you ever go to a gym! You can do the **Younger Body Now** routines in the comfort of your own home. I've already talked about how important strength training and cardio are. In the next chapters I am going to outline some workouts you can do at home. These will be based on the best exercises you can do and will prepare you for some more strenuous workouts in the future. The important thing is to start because basically anything you do at first – as long as you keep moving – is beneficial.

### The Beginners Approach To Cardio

Maybe you started walking ten minutes per day and you increased it five minutes per week. Lately you've been walking between 45 and 60 minutes per day. That's great! Now it's time to gradually increase the intensity. To do this we have to use a watch that has a second hand.

First, warm up with a 5-minute easy walk. Try and find a hill that you can walk up quickly for one minute. After a minute, stop and walk back down and then go up again. For the first time repeat this 4-6 times. Once you get in better shape, 6-8 times is optimal. This of course can also be done on a treadmill. Put the incline up high enough so you are working fairly hard for a minute. Then bring the incline down and walk easy from 1-2 minutes depending on how you feel.

This workout is also one that can be done if you run. I usually have my clients do a 5-minute slow jog for a warm up. After that, depending on their fitness level, I will start them at a level 5 or 6 incline at 5 miles per hour. The time spent running can be anywhere from 20 seconds to a minute depending on what kind of workout you want to do for that day.

After each interval we rest for 1 to 2 ½ minutes and I raise the incline by .5 and the speed by ½ mile per hour. We do at least 6-8 intervals, again depending on the fitness level. The total workout should take no more than 20 minutes. Interval training, as I have mentioned before, is much more effective in losing body fat and speeding up your metabolism because you are getting your heart rate up much higher than if you were doing a low-intensity workout. Your metabolism will increase the whole day and you will be burning fat because of it. If you want you could alternate a low intensity day with a high intensity interval day. For instance one day do a 3- or 4-mile walk or run and the next day do intervals.

Also when you are doing your interval workout you may want to use a heart rate monitor. I personally don't use one but they can be helpful to obtain your MHR (Maximum Heart Rate) as well as to see how many calories you burn. I try to get my clients' MHR close to 90-100% when performing their high intensity intervals. You can find your MHR by subtracting your age from 220. So if one of my clients who is 60 years old is doing a 30-second interval, their MHR would be 160 beats per minute. After the interval we would rest anywhere from 1-2½ minutes to get their heart rate back down. Taking your MHR is a good idea but I also have clients and athletes that don't take it. They let their bodies tell them when they are at the optimum intensity.

*Rev up your metabolism and burn fat all day.*

Track runners that are training for sprints or distance events all do interval training. Sprinters do shorter intervals such as 40-, 50- or 60- meter sprints then switch off to longer intervals, perhaps 100s, 150s, or 200s. Distance runners will do intervals ranging from 100 meters to 1500 meters.

One of my favorite interval workouts, which can be done on the track, open road, or field, is to run repeat 100s. I can do anywhere from 8-16 100s depending on how I feel or how much time I want to spend. After a 3- to 5-minute slow jog and 4-5 easy strides of about 40-50 meters, I am ready to go.

I start by striding the straights on the track and walking the turns. The straights are 100 meters and so are the turns so you are getting about 90 seconds rest after each 100 which is perfect. If I don't have access to a track I will estimate 100 meters by timing myself for about 20 seconds. I'll then walk for 90 seconds and repeat. If I'm doing 16 hundreds the first eight are usually slower strides to get my body really warmed up. The next eight are run much faster and the last two or three I try to sprint as fast as I can. The workout takes about 30 minutes including the warm up. At the end of the workout I know that I've had enough. I feel tired and exhilarated at the same time – what a great feeling!

Anyone can do the workouts at any level. After an easy warm-up you can stride real easy on the straights or road for 100 meters. (I prefer soft surfaces). Gradually pick up the pace on each one. Start by doing eight strides of 100 meters then add one stride each week until you reach the number you want to accomplish. You can also cut the workout in half by running the intervals faster.

One of my clients who is in her 70s had never run before so she started by running 30 steps. She gradually increased it to 50, then 10 meters and each time went a bit farther until she jogged for 100 meters. The point is anyone can start no matter what kind of shape you are in!

Another workout I like is to run stairs. If you don't have a stadium near you, there is always a set of stairs somewhere to run. They could be in your apartment complex, house, or anywhere you can find. It's a great way to get your cardio in, burn fat, and work your large muscle groups, quads, glutes, and hamstrings. Run or walk anywhere from 10-30 sets, depending on how long they are.

The point I am making is that there is no set time or distance, and it is up to you to make the intervals physically challenging. If you find that interval training is too demanding for you then go back to doing your lower intensity longer workout until you get in better shape. When the weather is cold I prefer working my clients out indoors or on a treadmill. The workouts last no longer than 20 minutes. After a 5-minute warm-up another example would be to jog 30 seconds and rest 1 minute. Each interval increases the speed and the incline. Usually 6-8 intervals will be enough.

## Strength Training – Short And Intense

A lot has been written about how long a strength training workout should be and how much time we should spend in the gym or at home. Through many years of training my clients, athletes, and myself, I have found that a shorter more intense workout is the best for overall fitness and conditioning. Also, a fast short workout burns more fat because you are always moving and there is very little rest between exercises.

From beginners to advanced, a shorter workout is most time effective. A longer workout is not necessary to achieve your goals. The only way I would train anyone differently in the gym would be if someone was just concerned about getting stronger on a certain exercise. If this were the case he or she would need a much longer rest period between sets (2-4 minutes) so the body is ready and rested enough to do a heavier set.

So by doing a shorter more intense workout of cardio and strength training, we are getting our heart rate up and burning more fat.

The 30-minute workout can be done anywhere from 2-5 days per week depending on your goals, the amount of time you have to spend, and how much effort you put into your workouts. The harder your workout and the more frequent your workout, the better the results you will get. Everyone can find the time they need to spend either at the gym or at home. You have time to start **to have a Younger Body Now**!

## Get On Your Bikes And Ride!

The workouts that we do walking or running can also be done on other exercise equipment. I personally like the bike because there is very little strain on the joints and for people that have had knee problems or arthritis it is an ideal way to get your cardio.

Most of us have done some recreational cycling before so riding a bike should be easy. You never forget how to ride a bike, right? There are two ways that you can cycle, indoors or outdoors. One of the negative points about riding outdoors of course is the weather. If it's raining you can usually take a short ride but riding outdoors in a storm is out of the question. Also riding during the cold winter months is nearly impossible, even for a die-hard cyclist like me. Having an alternative workout is a necessity and that is to ride indoors.

## Riding Indoors Or Out

If you belong to a gym your problems are solved. If you don't, you may want to invest in an exercise bike so you can ride at home. Also riding indoors is a lot safer than riding on the road. A nasty crash can keep you out of commission for a long time.

If you are going to ride outdoors a great place to do so is on trails in the woods. Since I am not competing in road races anymore I do all my riding on trails because it is much safer and a lot of fun. You have to have an off-road mountain bike to ride on trails. The added advantage is that you can ride it on the road as well. The fatter tires of the mountain bike make it an easier and safer ride.

There are usually a number of safe trails in your local and state parks that even a novice mountain biker can ride. There are books that list all the trails in most areas and you can also find them from a web search. Many urban areas have miles of greenways that are perfect for riding.

Once you become a more experienced mountain biker you can get clip-on shoes and pedals. They are designed to clip your feet into the pedals and unclip quickly, while giving more power and control to your cycling stroke. Also when you are going downhill in the woods, move your weight further back on the seat and use your back brakes instead of your front brakes to prevent you from flipping over the handlebars. It is also a good idea to bring a spare tube and small tire pump in case you get a flat. I also like to keep my tires fairly hard because this will help prevent a flat tire on rocky services. Experiment with your own tire pressure to find out what works best for you. Most importantly always wear a helmet. One time I flipped over my handlebars on a tricky steep downhill and my head hit a tree square on. That helmet saved my life and helped prevent many more serious injuries in my training and racing rides.

## Starting A Cycling Cardio Program

When you first start your cycling workouts you should go easy. Don't overdue it. You can start with a couple of easy rides or if you are on your exercise bike, spin easy for ten minutes. Since the bike takes a lot of pressure off your joints you can ride longer and farther than you could if you were walking or running. Another advantage of the bike is if you are running for your cardio and get injured, you can still bike and get the same cardio benefit.

## Options For Cross Training

Combining cycling and running is also a great way to cross train. One day you may want to ride your bike and the next day run. This is a great way to prevent overuse injuries because you are working different muscle groups on alternate days. When I was training for triathlons which incorporate running, cycling, and swimming, I got in really super shape.

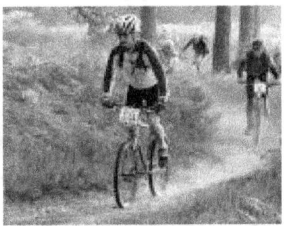

Riding your bike outdoors can give you a great interval workout by riding the uphills hard then coasting the downhills for recovery while spinning fast on the straights. You can also use your watch and time yourself for your intervals or pick a set distance to ride. For example you may want to ride as hard as you can for 400 meters, then ride real easy for a couple of minutes, then repeat. As in your running workouts you can pick any distance you want for your intervals.

When I bike indoors I usually spend no more than 30 minutes on the bike. I can pick as many intervals as I like for as long as I like. After a 5-minute warm-up, you can ride hard for 30 to 60 seconds then spin easy for 60 seconds. Repeat as many times as you like and try to keep the tension high on the intervals. Another workout would be as follows.

1.  5 minute easy spin
2.  1 minute fast spin
3.  1 minute recovery
4.  30 second hard hill (standing up)
5.  90 seconds recovery
6.  90 second fast spin
7.  2 minute recovery (riding easy
8.  60 second hill – 30 second on seat, 30 seconds off the seat followed by a 60 second fast sprint low resistance
9.  60 second recovery
10. 20 second sprint, 15 second recovery, 20 second sprint
11. 3 minute steady riding with medium resistance
12. 3 minute cool down

On the hills you can put the tension on the bike as high as you like but make sure it's not so high that you can't finish the interval.  Also getting off your seat when the resistance is real high will enable you to work different muscle groups, especially the glutes.  You can also do a fast sprint when you are standing up, (off your seat) when the resistance is low. This really gets the heart rate up!

You can do as many high resistance or low resistance (spinning) intervals as you like. Mixing it up will help prevent boredom.  I also find that listening to music during a workout makes the time go by faster and it's more enjoyable.

When I was a spin instructor I would do my intervals to the beat of the music.  When a slow song came on I would do a hard hill either seated or standing and when the music was fast it was time for a fast sprint. You can vary your whole workout to music if you like and just go with the tempo.

Keep in mind that when you are first starting out don't put the tension too high on the bike.  You want to get in better shape by strengthening your cycling muscles first. This may help prevent any knee problems in the future.

No matter what form of cardio you choose, walking, running, cycling, or swimming, if you make it an integral part of your life you'll never be sorry. The health benefits you get from the work you put into it will be more than worth the effort.

"I used to be in pretty poor shape. The thought of doing a 30-minute intense workout was unthinkable. Now after only six months, I not only can do the workouts, I have much more energy and my body has changed dramatically."

Andy Rothstein 59 years young

*7*

# Joining A Gym

## Now It's Time To Consider A Gym!

### Selecting the Right One

Now that you have gotten yourself on a daily routine of cardio and strength training, you can seriously think about joining a fitness center. Most fitness centers usually charge anywhere from $20 to $125 per month depending on what part of the country you live in. A lot of gyms charge more not necessarily because the equipment is better, but because of the extras they offer such as a better atmosphere, pool or spa, and fancier locker rooms. Usually a gym with the price range of $40 - $50 per month has all the basic equipment that you need.

In the cardio department, make sure you have the basic machines such as treadmills, bikes, and elliptical trainers. A good idea would be to see the gym during peak hours – or during the hours you will likely be going – to make sure there is not a long wait for a cardio machine. Some gyms put a time limit on their cardio equipment when it gets crowded.

Most gyms have the usual strength training equipment, pull downs, Smith machines, leg press, cable crossover, and a different machine for every body part. Of course you should make sure there are plenty of free weights and dumbbells.

### Picking the Right Trainer

Usually a trainer will show you how to use the equipment at least once and after that they want to sell you a training package. These training packages run anywhere from $35 to $100 per hour, again depending on what part of the country you live in. The more sessions you buy, the less money you are going to pay per session. If you are looking for a trainer remember that all trainers are not the same! First, try to observe some trainers working with their clients. So what are you looking for in a trainer? First we have to assume that all the trainers are certified, otherwise the gym would not hire them. Some gyms even put their trainers through their own certifications and train them extensively.

## She Is Your Trainer Not Your Therapist!

If you see a trainer that talks to his or her clients in between exercises for a long period of time, say more than two minutes, they are wasting the client's time and money. The workout should be flowing, going from one exercise to the next with very little rest. Too many trainers love to talk to their clients and tell them their life story. Of course the client does the same. The trainer turns into more of a therapist than a trainer because their clients may have no one else to talk to about their problems. It is really easy to become friends with your trainer but then half of your sessions will be spent talking rather than training!

I put my clients through a 30-minute workout and we keep moving the whole time. If we talk it is while they are doing an exercise. If you are going to get a trainer try and pick a gym that offers a 30-minute workout in their training package. In that 30 minutes you should be doing between 20 and 30 sets of different exercises depending on your fitness level.

*It's training, not therapy!*

## Does Your Trainer Look The Part?

When choosing a trainer make sure that he or she looks the part. In most cases a trainer that looks good and knows how to get himself in shape can get you in shape as well. I've seen so many trainers take some classes, study for the certification test, pass it, and suddenly they are a trainer! Certifications are certainly necessary and some trainers spend time getting certified in a number of areas. Usually if they take the time to study in their field they do become a better trainer. The person who has spent years getting him or herself in shape usually reads many fitness magazines because it is a way of life with them and they too make good trainers. Body builders, athletes, fitness competitors look the part and if their clients like the way they look they are an inspiration for them. Also these types of trainers usually have knowledge of nutrition because in order to get in that type of shape you must be able to eat well and diet for a competition.

## The Right Classes Are A Plus

Another thing to look at when joining a gym is to see how many classes are offered. Get your strength training in first, then your aerobics. You can even do your strength training and aerobics on different days but it isn't necessary. Taking some classes adds interest and variety.

Yoga classes are good for relaxation and flexibility, although they do very little for bone density or muscle strength compared to the weights.

Some other classes that I think are great are spin and body sculpt classes. Spin (biking) classes are a great way to get your cardio in. In spin you do all kinds of intervals on your bike while listening to music. You get hills, sprints, heavy resistance, spinning, and more.

A body sculpt class is usually strength training set to music. I've taken this class myself and feel it's a great way to do your weight workout. The class includes basic strength movements, squats, presses, and curls, all done to your favorite music.

So remember, if you are going to use a trainer, make sure that most of the talking is done while you are exercising and make sure your trainer looks the part! Consider classes after you've mastered the basics of a good workout.

If you can't afford a trainer don't worry, you will know the basic exercises from reading this book. This will be enough to get your own routines started. I've outlined the best exercises you can do at home. You can incorporate them into any routine you like.

## Nobody's Looking At You – Really!

Also don't feel intimidated by other people when you walk into a fitness center for the first time – or any time after that. For some reason people think that everyone is watching them when they go into a gym. This is probably true whether you are a male or female even if you feel you have a pretty great body. Actually, no one really cares what you look like. They're too busy trying to get themselves in shape. It's really easy to feel intimidated because after all we're all there to get a better body and to become healthier and fitter. We know we aren't in the best shape now so being somewhat self-conscious is totally normal when you work out. Even if I go to a new gym I feel that all eyes are on me and that people are judging my body even though I know I am in great shape.

For the average person it's not an easy thing to get enough nerve to join a fitness center, especially when it's your first time. Just remember everyone goes through the same experience. Actually my guess is that since a gym is all about bodies, it's natural to think that people would be looking at ours. When I see a person who is clearly overweight and out of shape in a gym, I say to myself how great it is that they are at the gym, trying to establish a healthier lifestyle. Give yourself a break too! You're showing your determination to live a healthier life by walking through that gym door.

In time everyone begins to feel at home in their fitness center as they become familiar with the staff and meet other members. Soon going to the gym will become one of the most pleasant experiences of the day. You will start looking forward to it more each day that you go.

*8*

## Results – What You Can Expect

### What Can I Expect If I Do My Part?

Now that you've joined a gym you should start feeling the results immediately.  If you have a trainer, he'll make sure your form is correct and also make sure that you get stronger and fitter with each workout.  If you are working out yourself, take care to try and add more weight to the exercises each couple of weeks and experiment with different types of equipment in the gym.

There are going to be days when you just don't feel like working out. You're tired or stressed out from work.  Maybe you have a headache or a slight cold and of course the most popular of all excuses, "I just don't have the time!"  That excuse always amazes me.  There is always time to work out.  If you get home from work late and you're tired, instead of taking a nap, exercise.  I guarantee you will feel a lot better after a 20- or 30-minute workout than if you took a nap for 30-40 minutes.  No matter how you feel I guarantee that when you are finished exercising you will feel better than before you started.  As I said earlier, my clients sometimes don't feel like coming in either but when they do, they are very glad they did.  Let your mind control your body. Remember, fitness is a state of mind.  You have already made the commitment, so stick with it.  No Excuses!

*Let your mind control your body because fitness is a state of mind.*

## The Results With Strength Training

## Strength Training Gets Respect

Strength training has come a long way in the past forty years. Back in the early and middle 60s only the hard core people worked out with weights. Everyone thought that lifting weights made you muscle-bound and athletes certainly would never consider the benefits of weight lifting. Today every sport from tennis, football, track, and even golf uses weight training to increase power, strength, flexibility, and physical conditioning. Now we know everyone can benefit from strength training. It's perhaps the greatest breakthrough to ward off the aging process and keep the mind and body younger.

Before all the scientific studies done on exercise and strength training we had no idea of the long term positive effects it would have on people. Of course there were famous people like Jack LaLanne who continued to work out as he got older but he was an exception, right? Well now we know that if we start to work out in our 30s, 40s, 50s, 60s, 70s, and 80s we can keep ourselves young. No matter when we start though we can reverse the aging process.

When I was in the gym business I trained many young people and some older ones to compete in sports and bodybuilding shows. I found that the over-50 crowd got the same results as the younger ones if they trained just as hard.

## But I Don't Want Big Muscles!

When I got the opportunity to train older clients in New York City I jumped at the chance. At first we started at their home but eventually we all joined a gym. The biggest problem I had to begin with was convincing the women to use heavy weights. They all had the idea that heavy weights would build big muscles. Of course I knew this to be false because I had worked with many women who lifted heavy weights and they never got bigger, they got tighter and firmer. Their bodies got smaller and denser. When you gain muscle you actually burn the fat and your body becomes smaller. Your body fat composition changes when you gain muscle so your percentage of body fat goes down. The more muscle we have the better our basal metabolism (the body's ability to burn fat when we are not exercising). After working with my clients for a couple of months I gradually incorporated heavy weights into their routine and their strength and fitness increased drastically. It didn't take years to get in shape and everyone got stronger and fitter each week.

So after 15 years of training what happened to the women that kept up their strength training? They are 15 years older but what about their body age? Let me give you some examples of the people I trained and the results they got.

## Some Client Case Studies

When Andrea first started working out with me she was 54 years old. She was in average condition for her age with very little stamina or strength. She said walking up stairs got her out of breath. I start everyone with the type of basic weight training exercises anyone could do at home. We had a bench, a barbell, and some dumbbells. I incorporated basic exercises that are still the most important to do in any routine you would do at a gym. I incorporated regular squats, lunges, bench presses, pullovers, pushups, all the best exercises you would do to change your body – but all at home.

Andrea got great results and so did everyone else I worked with. After a year we finally moved to a gym and incorporated the usual gym movements, heavy squats, leg presses, etc.

To everyone's amazement we kept adding more and more weight to our exercises and our group of 40- through 70-year-olds was soon leg pressing from 500 to 1000 pounds! Their bodies didn't get bigger, only stronger and fitter with increased bone density, ligament and tendon strength.

Andrea's endurance increased with her strength.  We began doing sprints, kickboxing, and even did a spot on CNBC.  Our workouts consisted of heavy weights, running short hills, stairs, 50- to 100-meter strides, and in the winter we did treadmill workouts instead of running outside.  Andrea is now 69 years old and she says her endurance is the best it has ever been in her life.  She can run up subway stairs without getting out of breath and the quality of her life is certainly better than the women her age who don't work out.

Another example of one of my clients who trained with my high intensity, fast-paced workout is 72-year-old Jackie.  At 72 Jackie is certainly stronger and fitter than she was 10 years ago.  Her balance has improved tremendously, along with her strength and endurance.  In one year she reversed the onset of osteoporosis from doing heavy weights.  Being so fit has affected her mind as well.  She thinks young because her body feels young.  Oh and did I mention that Jackie is a cancer survivor?

It doesn't take years to get a younger body.  I've found that most healthy people - no matter what the age - can improve their physical condition right from the start.

## Boomers Who Train Hard Get The Same Results As Their Kids!

Training people over 50 has been no different than training someone in their 20s or 30s.  The older athlete who works just as hard as the younger one gets the same results.  My conclusion is that if you take a person of any age, as long as they have no physical limitations, and train them as hard as any other athlete, they will all get the same results. Age doesn't matter!

One of my clients is a 65-year-old, very fit lawyer named Jeff. He started training with me when he was 58 years old.  He wasn't very strong or fit when he first started training and was your typical out-of-shape weekend tennis player.  At first the weights he used were very light but in a short period of time Jeff became stronger with each workout. Now at 65 years old he can do 15 pull ups, 50 pushups, and dumbbell press 70 pounds in each arm. Jeff says he is stronger now than he was when he was 25. His tennis game is amazing and he beats other men who are younger and were once tennis pros!

The one thing Jeff does that sets him apart from most men his age is that he makes his workouts top priority in his life. He is determined to get fitter and stronger as he gets older and every workout is a new challenge for him. He will actually leave a meeting so he doesn't miss a workout! To be super fit when you are in your 40s, 50s, 60s, and 70s, takes tremendous dedication and hard work. You can have a body age that is younger by 10, 20, even 30 years. Isn't that well worth it?

*Miss a meeting? Maybe, but never a workout!*

Of course not everyone wants to work that hard because they don't have as much drive or determination as some of my clients. The good news is that even with a moderate amount of work you will still look and feel younger and get great results. No matter how many hours or days a week you exercise it's still much better than doing nothing at all. Two days a week is good and more is even better. I have outlined your cardio workouts and given you the best strength training exercises to do at home with minimal equipment – there's no excuse not to start today!

I don't think there is anyone who started an exercise routine that didn't feel better afterward. You can't put a price on the health benefits you get after your body becomes younger and fitter. Mentally you can think better and more clearly. I've even had clients tell me they just feel "smarter"!

Physically of course we feel better, stronger, more energetic, less tired, and the quality of our life improves tremendously. One of my 52-year-old clients told me that her confidence at work improved so much that she started performing better and that landed her a raise!

## Bedroom Benefits Too!

Of course feeling less tired and more energetic has other benefits as well. Typically as we get older the desire and energy we have for sex seems to leave us. The older we get, sex becomes less important to us while other things like work, food, and even TV take up our time. Couples drift apart as intimacy decreases. It's easier to just roll over or fall asleep hugging the remote.

So why does having sex become less and less important to us? One of the reasons is that as we get older males and females produce less testosterone. It not only controls our sexual desire but the ability to perform as well. Testosterone is also the key hormone for building muscles and losing body fat and helps slow down the aging process.

Most of us have heard of hormone replacement therapy where synthetic testosterone is put into the body by weekly or monthly injections. Your doctor can tell if your testosterone level is low through a blood test but most men over 40-50 begin to have lower testosterone levels. Hormone replacement therapy is somewhat controversial and opinions vary. Testosterone is also the main ingredient in the anabolic steroids some bodybuilders and athletes use to get stronger and faster.

So what is the answer to our testosterone problem without putting it back synthetically? The answer is weight training. Strength training helps our bodies produce more testosterone naturally and also the fitter and stronger we are the healthier we become and the more we can look forward to doing more than sleeping in the bedroom.

Dr. Fred Hatfield, Co-founder and President of the International Sports Association suggests lifting weights increases testosterone levels[14]. Heavy weights with multiple sets using compound exercises such as squats and pressing movements spike testosterone levels in both males and females.

On the opposite side extreme endurance training like long distance running or prolonged aerobics could actually reduce testosterone levels, especially in males. Another reason for the short intense weight training and cardio workouts in our program! Short intense workouts will raise testosterone levels but longer workouts will not result in higher levels.

Besides weight training to increase our testosterone levels there are some supplements that could help us as well. A lot of athletes, including myself, take the amino acid Arginine. Arginine helps to produce nitric oxide which increases blood flow and helps our vessels open wider. It not only helps to increase strength and endurance but could be useful for erectile dysfunction because of the increased blood flow throughout the body. Also not all Arginine is the same and what seems to work the best is Arginine Ketoglutarate with added L Citrulline. The herb Tribulus Terrestris is used by some males to increase the production of testosterone. Two other supplements that may stimulate higher levels of testosterone are Fenugreek and Maca. Fenugreek works similar to Tribulus in raising Testosterone levels, and Maca helps the pituitary gland and endocrine glands to keep our hormones functioning normally. Another supplement that many athletes use to increase Testosterone levels and regulate estrogen levels in men is Nolvedex XT by Gaspari Nutrition. I have used this product myself and whether you are 30 or 65 years old it could certainly help to keep your hormones functioning properly. By combining weight training workouts with the right supplements we can not only increase our health and fitness but our bedroom benefits as well. Remember always consult your doctor before using any supplement, and take some time to research any product that you read about.

A couple of years ago one of my clients who was in his 60s told me that since he began working out his sex life with his wife had improved greatly. She also had been strength training. I told him that the increased level of testosterone from weight training was the reason for the renewed zest in his marriage! I have heard many other similar stories through the years, especially with my older clients.  A better quality of our intimate relationships is another great benefit we can get by taking the time to put strength training into our lives.  It is certainly better to increase our hormone levels naturally than to put a synthetic form into our bodies.

Just a few months ago Linda, one of my 76-year-old clients who had been training with me for ten years, came by.  She has maintained a great body as has her 81-year-old husband – also a client of mine – and I joked with her that her "glutes" looked great.  Not missing a beat she shot back with:  "Bill (her husband) thinks so too – we do it from behind!"  I had to laugh at Linda and Bill still enjoying a high quality of life and having the energy to enjoy loving each other.  Maybe that's what the "golden" years really mean!

## With Results Like These, What's Stopping You?

So why doesn't everyone start exercising?  There are many reasons: lack of discipline, poor motivation, lack of energy, insufficient desire, time, and career pressure.  Also a lot of people become set in their ways and just don't know where to start.  Hopefully reading this book will get all those who have never worked out before on the road to a younger body and all those who are working out now to improve as they get older.

Working out and becoming fitter is a great feeling. Sometimes I can't believe how many people miss out on this tremendous experience. Nothing feels better than finishing a great workout at the gym, working out at home, or going for a run or walk.  Your body and mind feel so alive and there is no better high in the world than that!

## Conquering Your Fears

I remember when I first started rock climbing with my son.  I had to overcome a tremendous fear of heights.  After I overcame that fear I really began to love the challenge that rock climbing gave me.

Sometimes it took every bit of strength that I had in my body to make it to the top of a hard climb but when I finished that climb the feeling was exhilarating.  The same thing happens when I have a great workout in the gym or when I'm running on the track.  There's no better feeling in the world to achieve something that we had to work so hard for.  I can see this same feeling that my clients get after working them out.  I guess that's one of the reasons they keep coming back for more.

""I used to work out with a trainer three times a week for an hour each time. With my schedule at work becoming more demanding I started the 30-minute workout and have gotten better results in a shorter amount of time."

Simona Stanica, 29

*9*

# Preventing Injuries

## Injuries Happen

No matter how old we are everyone, including the world's top athletes, has to deal with injuries. These injuries could come from the activities we are doing such as working out or playing a sport, or perhaps some unrelated reason. An injury could even come from the way we sleep – how many of us have woken up with a stiff back or shoulder pain? Athletes who are in great shape and train extremely hard are not immune to injury either and could lose a whole season of competition if they get hurt.

I have dealt with every type of sports-related injury with my clients and also myself. At some point anyone embarking on an exercise program will experience some type of injury. As a trainer I try to keep my clients from getting hurt but sometimes it can't be avoided. Sometimes our bodies can withstand a huge amount of stress and then suddenly we bend down the wrong way and our backs give out. Our knees are also very sensitive to injury and in a split second we can turn our leg the wrong way and suddenly we have pulled something.

I was training my son for the 200-meter sprint and he was in great competitive shape. One time after a race he tried to pull his shoe off with his other foot. Evidently he jerked his knee the wrong way and tore some cartilage and was unable to run for a year. All his racing and training and never once did he injure himself. One freak accident and he was out of commission.

The same is true for my clients whether they are 30 or 80. In one split second something goes wrong and an injury occurs. So many times I've heard my clients say that they woke up with some sort of pain. "My chiropractor said he thinks I did it exercising!" they tell me. No one knows for sure how an injury happened but I do know that it's impossible to avoid injury completely. Still we can take precautions to prevent some of them.

## Yes, Warming Up Is Important

First we must remember to warm up for whatever sport, workout, or event we do. If you're going to jog, walk for five minutes first. After that, start nice and easy and don't forget to do some light stretching. If you are going to do intervals, jog easy at first for about five minutes. After that, use the first four intervals as a warm up, starting out easy then picking up the pace gradually with each one.

If you're going to work out at the gym it's a good idea to start your workout with four or five minutes on the treadmill. When you start your weight workout do the first couple of exercises really easy and then gradually increase the weight until you are doing your maximum weight. If you are a beginner you're already doing light weights so you can get right into your workout after you do some light cardio.

## Oh, My Shoulder!

I find that the most common injury in the weight room is some sort of shoulder injury. If your shoulder gives you pain when you are exercising it could be a number of things. Tendonitis, or inflammation of the tendon, is one cause or you could have a tear in your shoulder or rotator cuff. The only way to tell for sure is to get an MRI and most of us probably won't do that. However if the pain persists I recommend going to your doctor or a sports medicine specialist to get it checked out. If my shoulder is in pain I usually try to ice it for about 15 minutes each night. I also take some ibuprofen every four hours to get the inflammation down.

After you get the inflammation down and the injury seems to feel better you can try to put heat on the area. Any product from the local drug store works. I like mineral ice for my minor pains. Usually heat warms the muscle up and if it's not a serious tear you can usually work out the soreness.

Another treatment that is worth looking into is Acupuncture. I have tried Acupuncture a number of times and found that it definitely helped my knee and shoulder injuries. My clients who have received Acupuncture treatments have experienced the same results. Anything is worth a try to alleviate the pain of injuries. Going to a chiropractor could also be beneficial. I know that many athletes, either on a world class or local level, go to their chiropractor to prevent and treat their injuries.

I personally like massage therapy because it gets the blood flowing in the joints and it's a great way to get rid of soreness and helps the muscles to recuperate after a hard workout or competition. Professional cyclists in the Tour de France get a massage every day after their race. Also track athletes and athletes from other sports use massage therapy as part of their training.

Another way to rehab injured muscles is hydrotherapy. If you have access to a whirlpool or swimming pool it will help a lot to ease sore and injured muscles. When you can't run because of an injury you can "run" in the pool since running is very effective in keeping your conditioning. No matter what you choose to help you recover from your injury, remember what works for some may not work for others. Do what works for you.

## Work Around An Injury

The bottom line is if it hurts don't do it!  I never stop working out completely if an injury occurs and I advise my clients to do the same. We should always try to work around our injury.  There are many exercises we can do that won't hurt us and that is one advantage of weight training.  If your shoulder hurts you can still work your legs, core, back, and arms.  If you have a leg injury you can still work your upper body.  If it hurts to run you can ride a bike.

There is a saying of "no pain, no gain" however if you feel pain that's a sign that something is wrong and you should stop and try something else.  If you have a knee injury I would lay off compound movements such as squats, lunges, and leg presses.  If you belong to a gym you can usually strengthen the knee area with some leg extensions.  I prefer to do them one leg at a time so you can tell when the injured leg is getting stronger.  I also like to take the supplement glucosamine sulfate for the joints which works particularly well on the knees.  It usually takes a couple of months to really work and I usually take about 2000 mg a day for myself. I recommend some other supplements for muscle or joint pain and injuries that I have found work for my clients and myself.  They are as follows:

Arnica Cream – sometimes helps muscle soreness

Super Cissus RX – could promote healthy joints, tendons and ligaments

MSM – might reduce inflammation of the joints and tendons

Bromelain – an enzyme that may help reduce inflammation

There are many other natural remedies to reduce inflammation and joint pain.  These are just a few worth looking into.

Remember when nagging injuries or pain persists, always get it checked out by your doctor so the problem can be diagnosed and treated.

"Since my husband and I have been doing Art's 30-minute workout our quality of life has improved dramatically. My knee problems have gone away and I can walk up and down stairs with no pain. My husband's back pain has also gone away."

Phyllis (67) and Monte (74) Morris

## *10*

# When It's A Matter of Life and Death

## A Chapter I Hesitated To Write

This is the one chapter that I hesitated to write because the subject matter is not very cheerful. However I thought it was most important because God forbid one of us has the misfortune to become sick. Hopefully leading a healthy lifestyle, exercising, eating right, and taking the proper supplements will help prevent us from getting any dread disease.

Through the years I have had clients who happened to have the bad luck of getting one form of cancer or another. I always told them to keep working out because it would keep their minds and body strong to help fight the disease. One man in particular brought this home to me, Lance Armstrong.

*With determination and drive you can beat the odds.*

Lance was the only person to win the Tour De France seven consecutive times and he was a cancer survivor. Being a competitive cyclist myself, I followed Lance's story from the very beginning of his great career. I remember reading his first book "*It's Not About The Bike*." The thing that impressed me the most about him was his determination and the drive that he had to beat the disease.

## Lance's Determination To Beat Cancer

When Lance was getting his chemotherapy treatments he would literally crawl out of bed and ride his bike every day.  It was only a 25 mile ride - nothing compared to his normal 100 mile training rides – but no matter how sick or tired he was he rode that bike. The other riders he rode with weren't near his competitive ability but in his weakened condition staying up with them was no easy task.  Perhaps it was Lance's mental toughness that helped him survive, along with his treatments and maybe just good luck. I'd like to believe it was just meant to be, so he could give all those people with cancer hope and the will to fight to survive.

I remember when Lance won his first Tour De France in 1999, everyone was surprised (except Lance). The French offered every excuse they could to make his win less magnificent.  After all, they said, some of the best riders in the sport weren't there that year.  Former Tour winner Marco Pantani of Italy and Germany's Jon Ulrich were missing from the Tour.  They eventually returned to the Tour and still Lance buried all his rivals year after year.

## Lance In The National Mountain Bike Championships

After his first tour win, Lance had made a commitment to ride in the National Mountain Bike Championships at Mt. Snow, Vermont. My son and I were also going to ride at Mt. Snow that year, Lance in the Pro division, my son in the Junior Sport and myself in the 45 and over class.  The course was a grueling six-mile loop with treacherous down hills and exhausting long uphill climbs.  The pro races were six laps of approximately 36 miles and my son and I had to ride two laps each. Let me tell you that those two laps were extremely difficult and grueling.  Lance's race was on Saturday and ours on Sunday and it was raining so the course was wet, slippery, and dangerous.

We got a chance to see the pros ride their race that day and I couldn't imagine how a road cyclist who was not an experienced mountain bike racer could possibly ride against the best pros in the U.S. Well Lance was in the lead for three or four laps and eventually finished in 6th place.  On that day my respect for Lance Armstrong grew even stronger. I never could figure out why the winner of the Tour De France would risk injury to ride in a mountain bike race when there was practically no financial award for him. Maybe after surviving cancer there was nothing in the world that he could ever be afraid of.

## My Son And I Finish Well

After four crashes and flipping over my handle bars twice on one of the treacherous down hills, I managed to finish 2nd in my race.  My son, who lost his seat on the 1st lap, continued to ride his race and still finished in the top ten.  Most riders wouldn't have continued to ride without a seat because it's nearly impossible to stand up on your bike for the whole race, but finish he did.

*After four crashes and a flip over the handlebars I finished second!*

As far as Lance goes, well the rest is history.  I watched every Tour De France that he raced.  When Lance initially retired from cycling so did I.  I know how much he inspired me and I can imagine how much he inspired people that have cancer.  Since Lance's retirement, he has run two NYC marathons and one Boston marathon, his best time being around 2 hours 48 minutes. The last two Tours had been uninspiring with drugs leading the headlines. In 2008 I cannot even tell you the winner's name because the tour just wasn't the same without Lance. As I predicted, Lance came out of retirement for the 2009 Tour de France, finishing well.

## My Client's Survival Story

About eight years ago one of my clients, Maria, who was about 58 at the time, was diagnosed with pancreatic cancer.  She was an avid strength trainer and runner and was in extremely great shape.  We both decided that she would continue her strength training even while she was getting chemo. During that time Maria never gave up hope. Even when she felt weak and ill from the chemo, she would still work out with me three times per week. She also continued her daily runs, but she toned down the intensity because her energy level was not up to par.

It was amazing that during this time Maria actually got stronger with the weights, not weaker. Psychologically this was a great advantage to her, and gave her both the physical and mental strength to fight the disease. Another interesting point is that the side effects from the chemo became less as she continued to train. Maria's frame of mind was very strong and she never doubted that she would beat the disease. Her positive attitude combined with her exercise routine and the treatment she was getting helped her recover.

Eight years later Maria is being trained by my son and continues to run and compete in road races, winning her age group in many of them. Like Lance Armstrong her will to survive and her determination to keep fighting and training helped her beat the odds. I have had other clients through the years that were stricken with cancer. I also encouraged them to continue their workouts no matter how bad they felt. Some worked out harder than others depending on how sick they were. The workouts helped them all, both physically and mentally. Thankfully all of them have survived.

*A positive attitude and the will to survive…*

## So What's Your Excuse?

I guess the reason I wanted to write this chapter was to inspire everyone – those with serious illness as well as those who are fortunate enough to be generally healthy – to realize there is really no excuse for not making exercise a part of your life. If people like Lance Armstrong and my client Maria can put aside the weakness, pain, and nausea of cancer treatments to fight for their lives, surely you can too.

"I had two major operations and I've always gotten my strength and muscles back with Art's 30-minute workout."

Elaine Housman, 69

## 11

# Filming The DVD

## A Picture Is Worth A Thousand Words

Over the years I have had the opportunity to train people from all walks of life and age groups. I don't think I ever thought that so many people, especially older people 50 and up, could get the results that they did. Writing a book was certainly one way to get the message out but showing it on film and hearing people talk about their experience was even better.

When I first got the idea to film a DVD for marketing purposes I knew that I had enough people to demonstrate the exercises. All the people we used for the filming were actual clients of mine and two other trainers who use my methods. One of my clients was a TV producer who, with his wife, had been working with me for about six months. They had gotten great results in that time so they totally believed in my training methods. When I told him what I wanted to do he liked the idea so we got a team together and organized the plan.

I wanted to have two people to represent each age group from the 20s to the 80s. These workouts were originally designed for any age group, not just people over 50 or 60. I wanted to show that someone who is 70 years old can do the same workout as a 30-year-old.

## Finding A Site

The next step was to find a gym that would allow us to bring thirty people, plus the film and sound crew, and film for eight hours in their fitness center.  We needed a place that had plenty of room to film the workouts, plus a quiet room for the testimonials.  One of my 52-year-old clients, Margaret, was going to leg press 900 pounds 10 times so I needed a real gym with good equipment.  My other two trainers, Lawrence and Cheyenne, all looked for a place in Manhattan, but it was much harder then we had anticipated so we had to look elsewhere.

Since I had family in upstate Kingston, NY I would travel there once or twice a month to get out of the city and spend time with my family. I worked out at a fitness center there called the MAC Fitness and felt it would be the perfect place for us to film. It was a huge facility with great equipment and the downstairs had a mini football and soccer field, sprint track, basketball courts and plenty of free weights. I knew the owner, Lyle Schuler, so I approached him with the idea.  He agreed to let us film there, so now I had to convince our producer to bring the film crew and the people participating two hours from New York City to the Mid Hudson facility. Since we had to pay the camera crew by the hour, we would lose four hours of filming time.  He finally agreed and the stage was set.

## Heading up to Kingston with my team.

The next step was to write a script for all the people that were going to demonstrate the exercises.  Since there were so many people we wanted everyone to do something different to keep it interesting.  Our age groups ranged from 23 – 83 years of age, showing that no matter how old you are you can still do the same thing that a younger person can do. I tried to put in a variety of challenges ranging from Olympic lifting, power lifting, and calisthenics, to kickboxing.

The shoot was to start at 9:00 am in the morning so everyone had to leave the city by 6:30 am.  I found it amazing that everyone was willing to give up their Sunday and travel two hours to be on film and not even get paid for it!  It showed me how much pride everyone had in themselves and how they wanted to show the world what working out had done for them.  Some had worked hard for months, others years, and now it was time to tell their story.

## Getting in front of the camera

The script was written.  The film and sound crew set up and we were ready to go.  As it turned out it was much easier to do a hard exercise in the gym then it was to do one in front of the camera!

We started the routines with my son Art, a 23-year-old All-American in track.  He did some Olympic lifts and pushups on two medicine balls while his feet were balancing on a stability ball.  The routine he did was extremely difficult and I had some of my older clients do the same routine. I wanted to show everyone that what we were doing had no age restrictions.  As we went through all the age groups it was obvious that all who were involved were in great shape.

My 71-year-old client Ellie performed numerous pushups and pull-ups and boxed with amazing form and power.  His boxing was certainly as good as the 31-year-old who performed the same routine. Then there was 76-year-old Ruth doing walking lunges with heavy weights at her sides, demonstrating balance, strength, agility, and flexibility.  Before she started working out she had to hold on to her husband while she was walking down the street because her balance was so bad.  Her husband Bob, 83-years-young himself, demonstrated his own strength by doing some heavy bench presses.  Bob had retired over ten years ago but since he started working out he began teaching at NYU and continues to do so to this day.

After lunch it was time for the testimonials so the film crew moved to another room. The testimonials took about two hours and everyone told their story of what it meant for them to be fit and feel so much younger.  For some it wasn't that easy to talk in front of the camera so the producer had to do two or three takes until he was satisfied with the results. After the testimonials everyone moved back downstairs to finish filming the exercises.

My 52-year-old client Margaret, who had been practicing for months, leg pressed 900 pounds ten times.  Everyone went through all their routines, excited that the work they had put in for months and years was going to be shown on film.  These athletes did a great job in showing their strength, fitness, and athletic ability.  It proved that when you put your mind to it and work out the right way, anything is possible.

## The Pride of Accomplishment

All in all it was a great day and the filming of "Younger Body Now" was a success.  Even though there was a lot of waiting around during the day, we had very few complaints and everyone enjoyed the experience of getting together to show what they could do.  Everyone was supportive of each other which brought a feeling of pride and unity between the younger and older clients.  After everyone left, the producer filmed Lawrence, Cheyenne, and I working out with our own routines.

The day was done and the "Younger Body Now" filming was finished. We were all very satisfied with the way the day went.  To me and the other people involved it was proof of what strength training can do at any age.  With the exception of my son who is an All-American sprinter, all the people involved were average, everyday, people with no athletic experience or background.  It was exciting to see people in their 40s, 50s, 60, 70s, and even 80s at the top of their game – the game of life.

# *12*

## The Mind-Body Connection

### Exercise Is Habit Forming!

Starting your exercise program once you have made the commitment to do it is the easy part.  Staying with it is going to be the hard part. As I mentioned before your mind has to take control of your body or your body will give you every excuse in the world not to exercise that day.  Remember most of us live our lives by habit – both good and bad. We have a habit of eating certain foods, we smoke, drink, go to church on Sundays, the list is endless. Exercising has to become almost like an addiction if we are going to stick with it for the rest of our lives. Developing the exercise habit is going to be the most important thing that you could ever do.  Because it is a positive habit, it will add many more quality years to your life.

*Excuses, Excuses, Excuses!*

I will list some of the excuses we are all going to use at one time or another. Of course at times there will be a valid excuse to cancel your workout for the day.  The bad part is you might be tempted to use one of these excuses every day of the week!

Here are the "Top Ten" reasons to skip exercise:

1.    I'm just too tired today.
2.    I don't have the time right now.
3.    I'd rather do something else (e.g. go shopping, catch a movie).
4.    I'm feeling depressed.
5.    I just don't feel well today.
6.    Visitors are arriving from out of town.
7.    My spouse won't go.
8.    The kids need me.
9.    I have to work late.
10.   My favorite TV show is on.

The list is really endless, but I'm going to try and address a few of these excuses so we have the tools to fight back when they come up.

Everyone at some point in time is going to feel tired before they work out. We have to remember that afterwards *you will always feel better*. So many times I just wanted to stay home and relax but I knew that after that workout I would feel fantastic. The same is true with all my clients and it will be the same for you.

You have to work around your excuses. There will be times when you don't have enough time to go to the gym because you worked too late or you have to stay home because of your spouse or kids. Then it's time to use some of the routines at home that we have put in this book. Anyone can get a great workout in 15 or 20 minutes if the intensity is high enough. I can put myself through a 15-minute workout at home and if I push myself hard enough, that's all I need.  You can do the same.

*No excuses!  Your health is too important.*

A lot of my clients call me and say they are sick and ask me whether or not they should come in to work out. I usually tell them if they have a cold to come in for an easy workout. Of course if they are really sick in bed with a fever I tell them to stay there!  Having a slight cold should not prevent you from working out and it will actually make you feel better afterwards.

When I have clients who have friends in from out of town I tell them to bring them along to the gym. Let them watch or do some light cardio. They might even get inspired to start on an exercise program themselves. If I have friends that are visiting for the weekend, I'll always make the time to go out for a half hour interval workout and they never seem to mind.

We have to make working out a habit and not let any excuse get in the way.  Probably one of the hardest things to overcome is depression. When you're feeling depressed you don't want to do anything, much less exercise.  We all get depressed in our lives. It's something that nobody can escape. Things like finances, a bad relationship, or a death in the family happen to us all.  We even get depressed because of the way we look or because of poor health. The list goes on. I'm not a shrink so I won't analyze all the causes of depression but I do know that the best thing to do when you are depressed is to work out. Even your therapist would agree with that since exercise has a significant and positive impact on mood. Afterwards suddenly that dark cloud above us is lifted a little higher and we feel much better.

*Exercise:  good for the mind, the body, and the soul*

There is a growing body of research that shows that exercise can be just as effective as drugs for depression. Exercise reduces irritability, fatigue, and self doubts and boosts confidence[15].  An October, 2007 Mayo Clinic article says that even 10 – 15 minutes of exercise give a temporary boost to your mood. Thirty minutes 3-5 times a week can significantly reduce symptoms of depression. The Clinic recommends that you set a reasonable goal to get yourself started, think of exercise as a tool to help you feel better, and get rid of what's stopping you from starting and sticking with your exercise program.

Researchers at Duke agree that exercise can be used to treat depression[16]. They report a 1999 study that showed many depressed patients improved through exercise alone. The effects seemed to be even greater in older patients.  No matter how bad things seem, getting your body moving will improve your outlook and ability to cope with the stresses of life.

One of my clients whose father was dying told me that she was by his side day and night because his time was near. She said that every day she would do a 30-minute workout and it gave her the physical and mental strength to deal with the stress. Exercise releases endorphins in the brain – those "feel good" chemicals - and we actually feel elated when our workout is through.

I always try to tell my clients to appreciate the positive things they have in life and not focus on what they don't have. If we are alive and healthy today and feeling good that's a lot to be thankful for.  So many people are less fortunate than we are and will never have a chance to develop and experience really good health.

**The Mind and Body Connection In Athletics**

Let me give you a few examples of the mind body connection in sports. We know that genetics play a large role in any sport. Some people are just born with the genes to be faster and stronger than others. Some will have more natural endurance, others will be thin no matter what they eat, while others will have to work very hard to keep their weight down. However if you work hard and know what you are doing you can improve on what your genes have provided.  The mind plays a major role on how those genes get expressed in your everyday life.

*Your genes get you started.  Your mind does the rest.*

If you have two athletes who are training for a sport whether it be running or tennis and they both have the same genetic makeup and work equally hard, who is going to be  the better athlete?  The athlete with the stronger mind will be the winner. An athlete has to have the proper mindset from the beginning of his or her career. He or she has to give 100% to their training and nutrition and with the right coaching they will succeed.

When an athlete competes, his mind has to be in control of his body from the beginning of his training to the day of his competition. He doesn't miss a workout for any reason because he knows the only way to make it to the top is to put in 100% effort.

*A stronger mind beats a stronger body*

When I am doing an interval training workout on the track and I'm trying to run 10x200 meters in 29 seconds with a 2-minute rest in between, I have to be totally focused on what I want to accomplish. After the 6th 200-meter interval my body says it's too tired to run the next 200 in 29 seconds because it hurts too much! That is when the mind takes over and pushes the body to finish the workout.

During a race or any athletic event the same thing happens to an athlete. When the body gets tired and wants to ease up, the mind has to take over. The same thing is true for someone who is just starting to exercise. Your mind has to control your body. If you want to reach your goals and attain a high level of fitness you have to overcome the feeling of giving up just like an athlete does.

Just the other day I was talking to one of my 62-year-old clients who has been with me for about eight years. He said that in the past it was a struggle to come to his workout because he had every excuse to cancel. Now he says he never thinks about canceling. He has trained his mind to overcome his body's desire not to work out and it has become a habit to come to the gym.

## Just Do It!

We've all heard the expression "just do it."  Like my 62-year-old client who never thinks about canceling anymore, we can't make working out a decision-making process.  We just have to do it.  Sometimes in life we want to do something that we've never done before but we hesitate because something in our minds makes us afraid.  It might be skiing, joining a gym, learning to swim, skydiving, etc. but we put it off and it never happens.  I think of the phrase "just do it" when it comes to doing something I want to do or planned on for the day. If the weather is cold outside and I have a run planned I don't think about whether or not I will run, I just do it. We have to put that phrase in our minds when we are planning to exercise. No excuse, no decision, nothing to think about, just do it.

*Forget about yesterday and tomorrow.*

## Your Workout Time Is Your Time

Another expression I like is "being in the moment." We've all heard the expression but what exactly does it mean? My definition is that there is no past, no future, only being and feeling in the present time. When we work out, we focus on every repetition of every exercise we are doing, trying to get good form and pushing ourselves to complete the set. Our mind thinks of nothing else during our workout, the rest of the day has left us, and for that 30 or 60 minutes, all of life's problems and hassles are gone. What a great way to get rid of stress. We push ourselves hard, to our utmost limit, we struggle, we sweat, but we love it. For that time when we are running, or cycling, or in the gym, is our time and no one else's. We control that time when we are working out or playing our sports and that helps us control all the other aspects of our lives.

*Any day you work out is a good day!*

I work out every day, not just to get fit and look good, but for myself. No matter what happens that day, if I work out, it's a good day. Other people that work out experience the same feeling of accomplishment and satisfaction that we get from reaching our goals, getting stronger, fitter, and looking better.

Sometimes I think about how so many people never experience that great feeling you get from feeling really healthy and fit. What a high it is being alive, healthy, and strong! Too many people live each day just getting older and more out of shape, their minds becoming stagnant.

Some of you reading this book will start an exercise program and will relate to everything I am talking about. There will be others who will start but not continue and still others who won't start at all. For those of you who do start it will be a big mental relief to know that you are finally doing something about your health. My clients know that working out and staying healthy is the most important thing in their lives. For those of you who read this book and change your lifestyle forever, it will be the same for you.

What a high it is, being alive, healthy, and strong!

# *13*

## A New Breed of Athlete

### No Limits

There's a new breed of athletes competing on the sports scene these days and they're here to stay. They have been around for a while but their numbers are growing rapidly every year. From all over the country, even the world, they're changing the perception of aging forever. They compete in every sport from football, hockey, track and field, cycling, gymnastics, and tennis to bodybuilding, just to name a few. They are the over-50 crowd, the baby boomers and beyond, people in their 50s, 60s, 70s, 80s, and 90s who refuse to let age stand in the way of competing in the sports they love. They lift weights, do interval training, and practice hard for their sport. They are the true warriors of the day.

Their competitions are on a local, state, national, and world level. Age groups can start at 40 and go up in 5-year increments until, well let's just say there are no limits! Each state usually has its own competitive games and national qualifiers and there are different sanctioning organizations in most sports. There are the Senior Games which start at 50 and over. Each state will have the games in a different county or city each year. Every other year is usually a National qualifier and the top two athletes in each of their events get to compete in the Nationals. These athletes take their sports very seriously and train extremely hard to be the best they can at their game.

Most states have their state games for all the age groups such as the Empire State Games in New York State, and include a Masters division which usually starts at age 35. Both men and women compete in their age group and every five years they look forward to moving up to compete in a different age group. Getting older to this group just means more fun! Most sports in the senior and state games are well represented and there is usually something for everyone.

## The Sport of Bodybuilding Grows

A sport that is growing at a very fast rate for men and women is body building. We all know that as we age our bodies begin to sag and we lose the tightness in our skin that we had when we were younger. Bodybuilding is a sport that judges you just for your look, so when you're up on stage with your skimpy posing trunks in front of a large crowd, you better look the part. It's amazing that people in their 60s, 70s, and 80s are up on stage, proud to show the bodies they have worked so hard to get.

I have competed in many shows on a local and national level. It takes much discipline to train and diet to be able to get up on stage and compete with the best. You lift weights, do your cardio, practice your posing, stick with your diet, all leading up to that one day of competition. Usually it takes about three to four months of dieting to get your body fat down to a very low level. To get rid of water weight, all carbs are cut out a week before the show. The last couple of days you start eating a lot of carbs again to give the muscles a fuller look. The night before the show is spent painting yourself with a product called Pro Tan. You try and get yourself as dark as you can because the bright lights on stage will hide your muscle definition. Three to five coats usually works very well but in the morning another coat is necessary because a couple of coats are left on your bed sheets!

Competing in the show itself is physically hard and demanding on our body. Dieting has left you a little weak and perhaps you cut out your water intake to get the muscles even tighter. The afternoon show is the prejudging and that's when all the competitors will do the mandatory poses together. Most organizations pick the winner from the afternoon prejudging while the evening show is for the crowd. Each competitor goes on stage and does his own posing routine to music which lasts anywhere from 60-90 seconds.

Most bodybuilding organizations have contests that have Master's Divisions for over 40-, 50-, and 60-yr-old athletes. The NPC (National Physique Committee), one of the largest organizations in the country, has a National Masters competition for bodybuilders over 40. The competition is tough and everyone - age 40 – 80 - looks great.

## My Competitions

When I was 40, I competed in the NPPC, Natural New York City Bodybuilding Championships. I came in 2nd place to a 72-year-old body builder. That same year I came in 2nd place in the 40 plus class in the Natural USA Bodybuilding Championships, go figure! A recent New York Times article, "60 Plus Ripped and Natural", stated that in the last five years the number of men and women in their 60s and 70s competing in U.S body building federation shows has doubled[15]. (New York Times Thursday, April 3, 2008, Abby Ellin) The Fame World Tour, which is a series of physique competitions founded by Jeffrey Kippel for the 60-plus division, drew enough contestants that Mr. Kippel's organization hired Scot Hults, a retired naval officer turned bodybuilder, to be in charge of the 60-plus division. "Age is a statistic, not a burden and there is no reason a man or woman can't get into and maintain the best shape of their lives at any age." Hults commented.

These bodybuilders have the same training principles that I advocate for my clients: hard workouts, a great mental outlook, and the right nutrition plan.   Vitamins plus supplements recommended by Dr. Antonio, chief executive of Internal Society of Sports Nutrition, include creatine for strength, glutamine for muscle recovery, and branch chain amino acids for muscle development.

When I was training clients for bodybuilding shows, diet and supplements were of the utmost importance for losing body fat and gaining muscle. You also have to have the confidence to know that if you do everything you are supposed to do you will be ready to compete on the day of the show. The seniors who compete in their sports all have the confidence and zest for life to achieve their goals and they don't let aging stop them. We're not all going to compete in the master's division in bodybuilding or the Senior State Games, but we certainly can compete with ourselves to get healthier, fitter, and stronger, and to have a greater quality of life for as long as we can.

*14*

## Starting Your Own Program

### Now It's Time For You To Get Started!

OK, so you've gotten the go-ahead from your doctor and now it's time to get down to business!  The only equipment you are going to need is a chair and a set of dumbbells.  If you are just starting out a set of 3- and 5-pound dumbbells will be enough.  If you have worked out before you can start with the 5s and go as high as 25 or 30 pounds in 5-pound increments depending on your fitness level.

I'm going to illustrate all the exercises you can use in your workouts. The routines you can use will be broken down into an "A", "B", or "C" workout.  An "A" routine will be easier to do than a "B" or "C" routine because the exercises are basic movements and easier to do.  However even an advanced athlete could do an A routine and make it intense. You can follow the routines exactly as I present them or you can mix and match and develop your own workouts.

If you have never worked out before you can start by practicing each movement in the illustrations for your first A workout.  The workout should take anywhere from 15 to 30 minutes. Take as much rest as you need between exercises and start out slowly. Let's get you on a 2- or 3-day a week program at first and alternate this with your cardio workouts. Remember cardio is important so you should be walking as much as you can, time permitting.

Our ultimate goal is to do a 30-minute workout, moving from each exercise to the next with very little rest. This will keep your heart rate up and burn the most calories and fat. Remember if you are first starting you shouldn't push yourself to the point of feeling exhausted. If you have been exercising already you can move through the routine at a faster pace, doing anywhere from 20 to 25 sets in 30 minutes.

When you are just starting out if you don't feel comfortable using your 3- and 5-pound dumbbells, just use your own body weight. After a couple of workouts or when you feel ready, incorporate the dumbbells into your routine. If you have already been working out you can use as much weight as you like. The goal is to use progressively heavier weights and perform each exercise almost to failure. "Failure" means the last repetition is extremely hard to do and one cannot physically perform another one.

I also want you to get yourself a notebook and record each exercise you do, the number of repetitions, how much weight you are using, and how much rest you are taking between each exercise. You are going to start with ten repetitions on each exercise. Try and use a two-second count on the positive movement and a four-second count on the negative.

When you strength train you have to remember that it's not about getting the weight from point A to point B. It's about really feeling the muscle you are working as you get from point A to point B. That's the reason I like to perform the two- and four-second count on each exercise. Slow controlled movements with very strict form and no swinging or momentum to get the weight up are the proper way to perform each exercise.

For the first A workout I have selected basic compound exercises and the ones that I feel are the most beneficial to start. You are going to do one exercise for each individual body part for ten repetitions to start. Perform each movement once then to go the next exercise. After you have finished all the movements, rest three minutes and do them again if you have the energy.  You can do anywhere from one to three circuits (see the complete set of exercises).

"There is a fountain of youth. It's called exercise!"

## 15

## The "A" Workout –

1. Warm up

2. Squats

3. Two Arm Dumbbell Press

4. One Arm Dumbbell Row

 5. Modified pushup

6. Plie' Squat

7. One Arm Tricep Extension

8. Crunches

9. Dumbbell Curls

**Ten Repetitions Each Exercise, Brief Rest Between**

1.  Warm up with some easy arm swinging.  Perform the 1st circuit using a very light weight to warm up.
2.  Squat – no or light weights, arms at your sides.

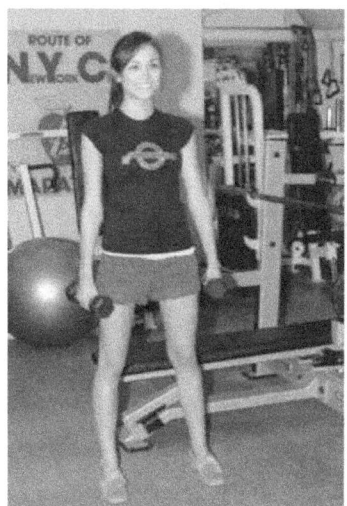 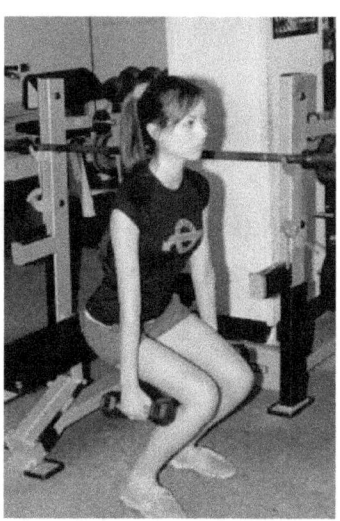

Start in the standing position and hold two dumbbells at your side. Use any weight that you can comfortably do for 10 repetitions. You may want to start with no weight if this is your first time. As you lower your body, lean back as if you were going to sit in a chair. Keeping your feet firmly on the ground with your weight more towards your heels than your toes, lower yourself to the position you see in figure 2.  If you cannot go that deep, go as low as you comfortably can. Try and use slow and controlled movements with a 4 second count on the way down and a 2 second count on the way up. Squats are the #1 glute exercise and they also work the hamstrings and quadriceps. Since you are working the largest muscle groups in the body, squats also burn the most calories and are great for cardio as well.

### 3.  2-arm dumbbell press – Shoulders

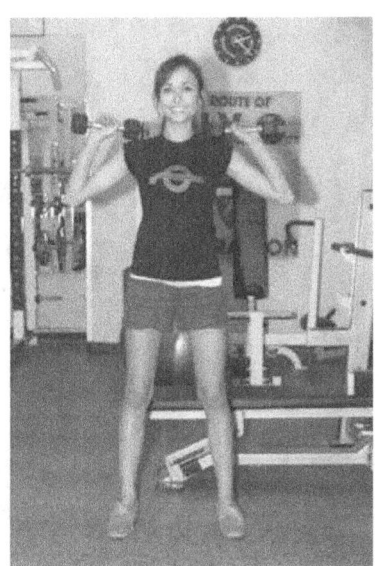 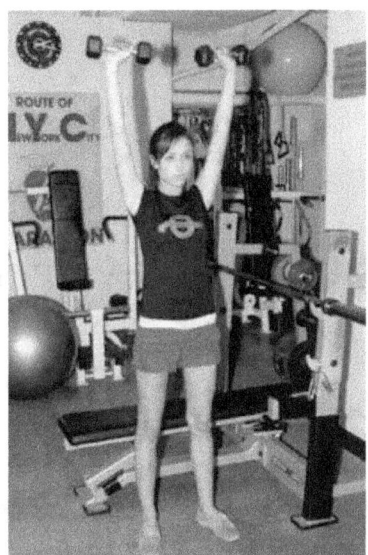

You can pick a fairly light weight on this exercise. If you are a beginner, 3-5 lbs are probably enough. If you have worked out before, 8-10 lbs might be more in your range. Start with two dumbbells on your shoulders and press the weight to the overhead position; using the 4 second up, 2 second down count, keep your palms facing away from your body as show in the illustration. Perform 8 repetitions to start and when you are ready for your second or third circuit, try to use heavier weights.

## 4. 1-arm dumbbell row – Back and arms

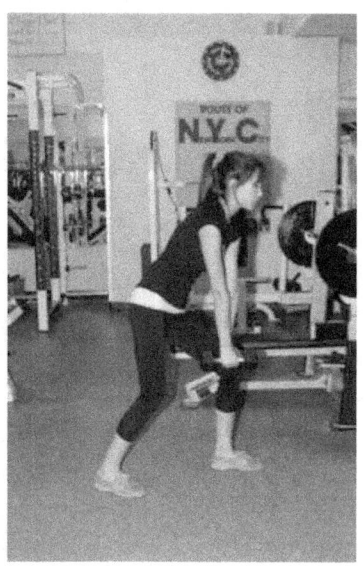 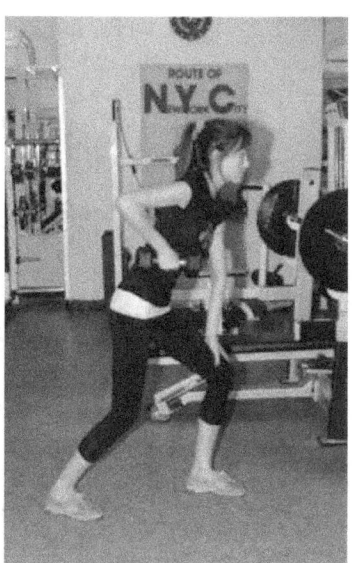

Use a heavier weight than you did on the dumbbell press. A 10 lb dumbbell should be enough if you are a beginner and a 15-20 lb dumbbell if you have worked out before. While leaning forward, place your left hand on your left leg, let your right hand hang to your side as shown in Figure 1. Bring the dumbbell in a controlled manner until the top of the dumbbell touches your chest. Lower slowly and repeat 8 times. Be sure to get a stretch at the bottom of the movement.

## 5. Modified pushup – chest shoulders and triceps

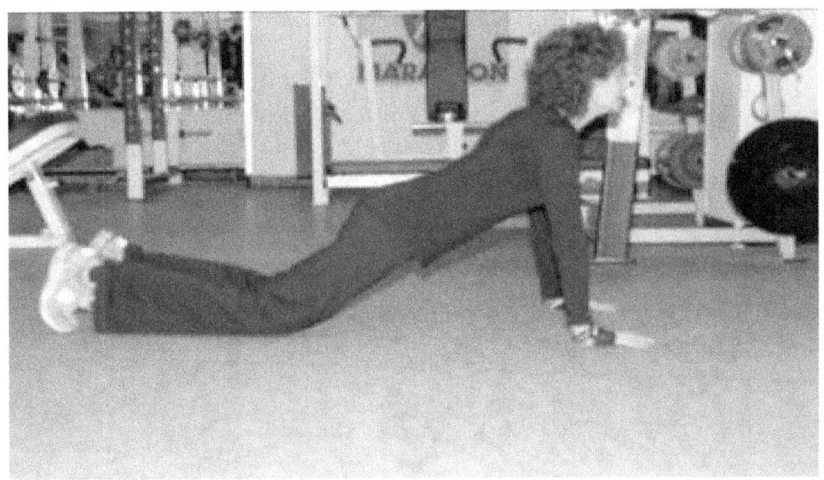

Start in a kneeling position with your hands shoulder width apart. Try to keep your knees as far back as possible, see illustration. While keeping your head up, put your elbows in an outward position and lower your body as low as you can and return to the starting position. The stronger you are, the lower you will be able to go. You may only be able to lower yourself a few inches at first, but your goal is to get your chin as close to the floor as possible. When you can perform 20 modified pushups in good form, try to do a few regular pushups. Only go down a few inches at first, and as you get stronger gradually lower your body closer to the floor.

### 6. Plie' squat with dumbbell –Inner things, quadriceps, glutes

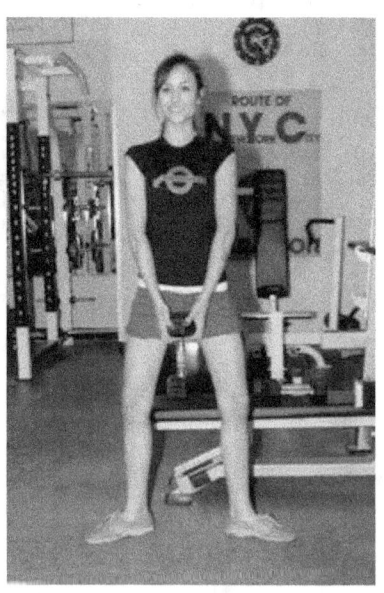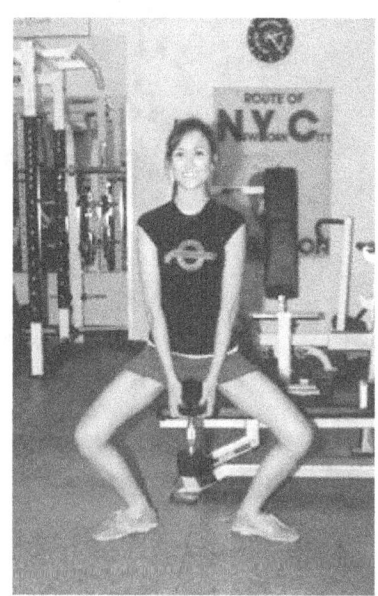

Start in a standing position, holding the top of the dumbbell in front of you. Unlike the regular squat where you sit back and lower your body, in the plie' squat you keep your body straight and lower the dumbbell as close to the floor as you can. Your feet should be about 18 inches apart and both feet are turned out to the sides. Ten repetitions is your goal to start and you should gradually increase the weight.

### 7.  1-arm triceps extension

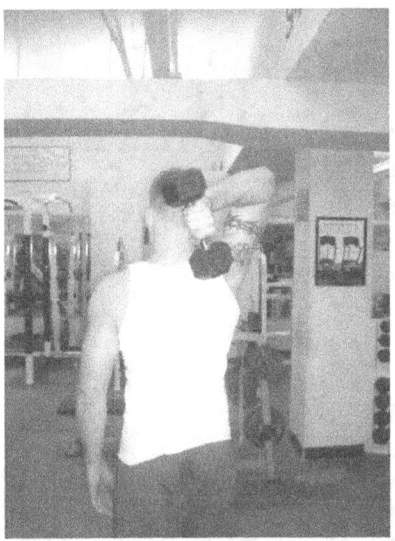 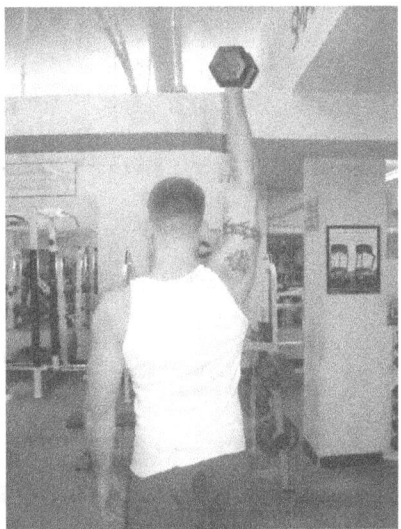

This is an isolation exercise that only works the triceps and does not incorporate another muscle group. Start with a light weight 3-5 lbs. With your right arm, push the weight overhead, keeping your arm as close to your ear as possible. Lower the weight as far as you can, and come back to the starting position.

## 8.  Crunches - Abdomen

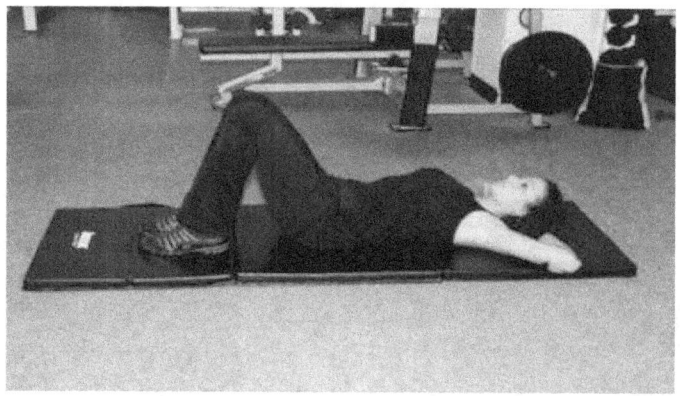

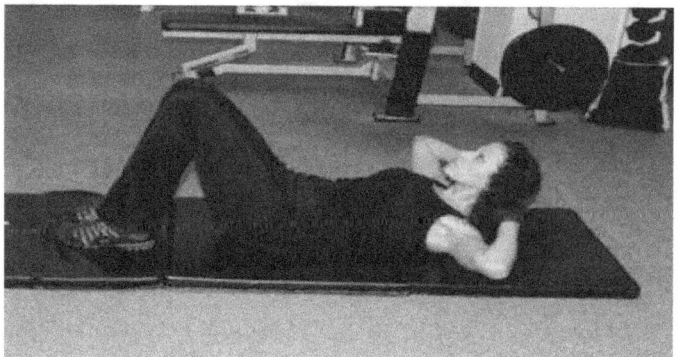

Lie flat on the floor, hands behind the head, knees bent. While keeping your chin on your chest, use your abs to pull your head and shoulders about 10 inches off the ground. Keep your lower back on the floor. Perform 20-30 repetitions.

### 9.  Dumbbell curls – Biceps

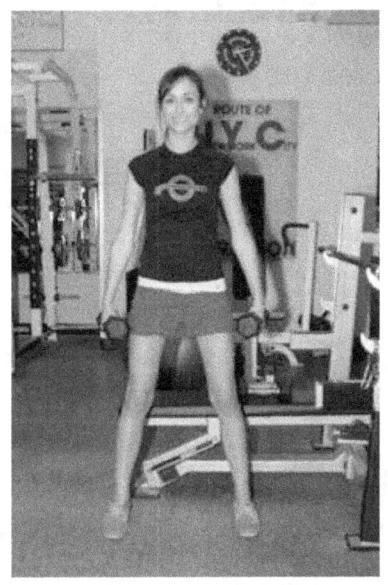 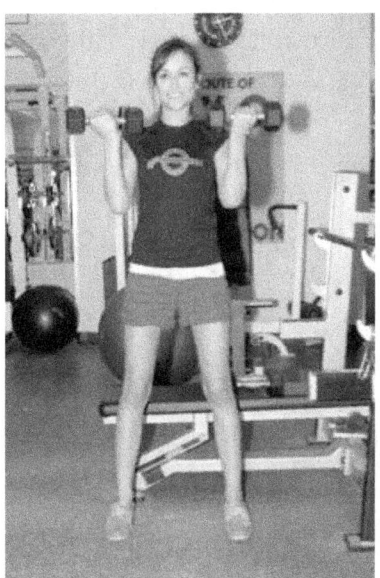

From the standing position take two dumbbells and hold them at your sides. Curl both arms up into the position shown in Photo 2. Perform a 4-second count on the way up and 2-second count on the way down. Start with a light weight of about 5 lbs, more if you're not a beginner. Add more weight when you feel the weight you're using is not challenging enough. It doesn't take long before you become stronger so continue to increase the weight and move from one exercise to another with less rest in between.

If you are going to do a 2nd circuit and you used 3-pound dumbbells on your 1$^{st}$, raise the weight to 5 pounds on each exercise.

After you have been on the 1$^{st}$ A circuit for two weeks or more, you can try the 2$^{nd}$ A workout. I have added a few more exercises for the second routine. Remember any A, B, or C workout can be very hard if you make it that way, however it's always good to add variety to your routine and work the muscles from different angles.

## Second "A" workout

1. Jumping jacks

2. Squats, dumbbells at sides

3. Alternate dumbbell press

4. One arm dumbbell row

5. Plie' Squat

6. Side Laterals

7. Crunches – feet up

8. Alternate dumbbell curl

9. Chair dips

10. Bent-leg dead lifts

11. Leg Raises

## Continue ten repetitions with brief rest between each set

1. Jumping Jacks to warm up. Perform lighter weights on the 1st circuit. Try and perform two circuits using heavier weights.
2. Squats (dumbbell at sides) since the legs are a large muscle group you can use much heavier weights then the upper body movement.

Use the same form as you did in the first A workout. You should be in much better shape if you have been performing this exercise for 2 to 6 weeks. Start using heavier weights. You can even increase the number of repetitions to fifteen.

### 3.  Alternate dumbbell press

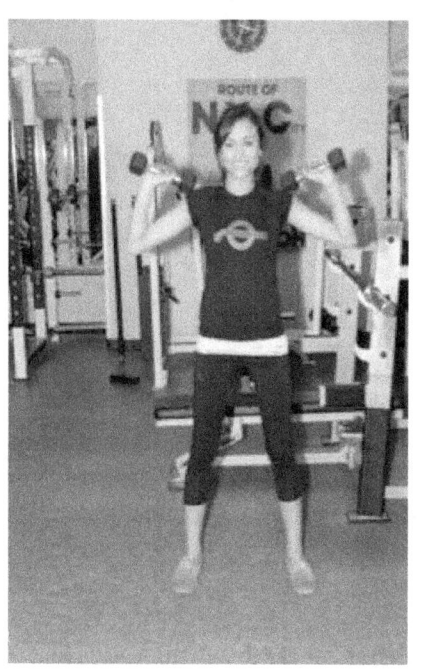 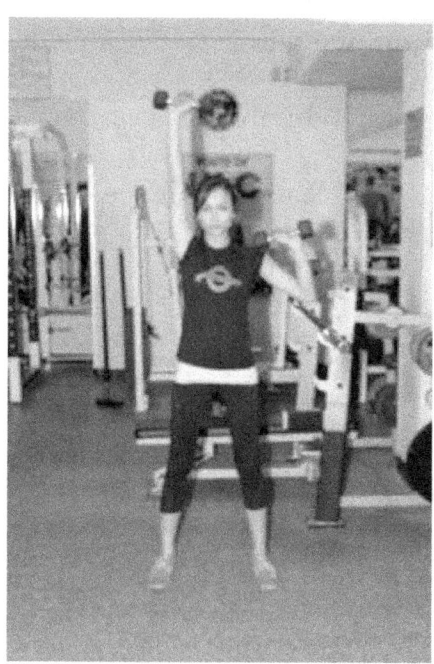

The alternate dumbbell press is similar to the two-arm dumbbell press. The difference is you are going to press your arms one at a time.  Using alternate arms is a great way to focus on each arm individually.  Start by pressing the right arm straight over head and making sure to keep the arm as close to the head as possible (see Photo 2).  When you get to the top, lower the weight to the start position (see Photo 1). Immediately press the left arm up using the same form.  Do not move both arms at the same time and always keep one arm at the starting position. Do 8-10 repetitions.

### 4.  One-arm dumbbell row

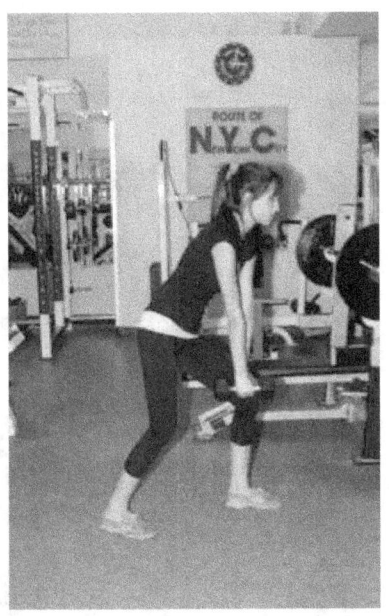 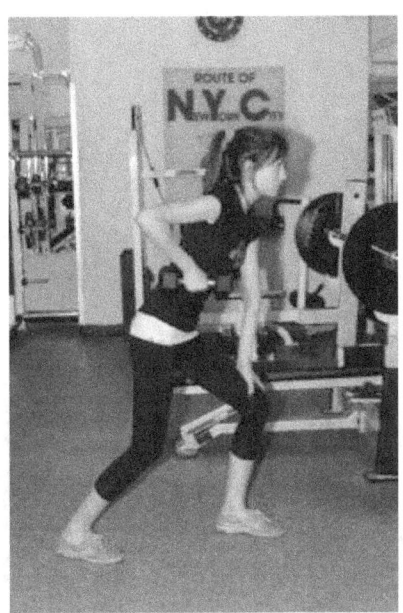

Use the same form as the A workout.  Since the back is a large and strong muscle group, you can use a fairly heavy weight.  For example, if you are using 10lbs on the dumbbell press you should be able to use 20lbs on the dumbbell row.  If you are using 5lbs on the dumbbell press you should be using 10lbs on the dumbbell row.  Do 8-10 reps.

## 5.  Plie' squats

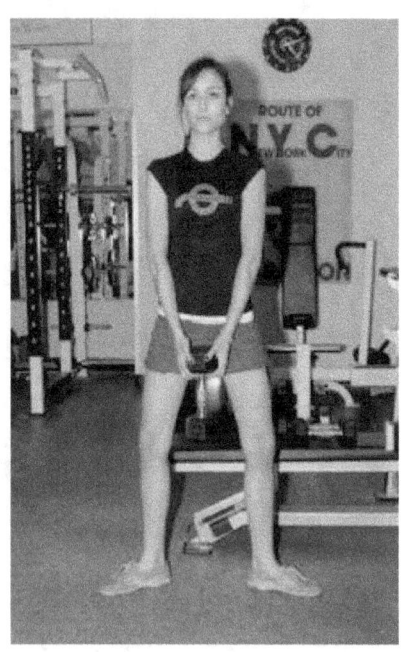 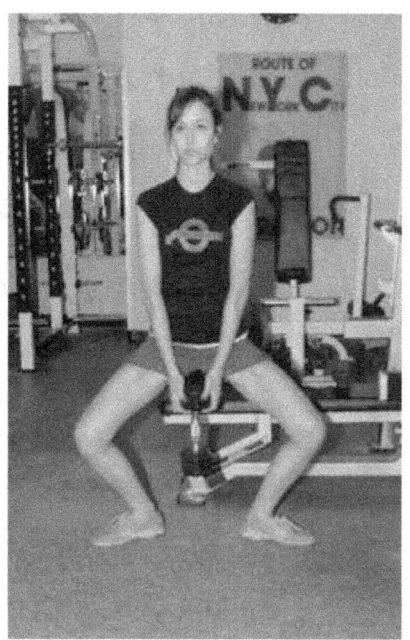

Use the same form as the A workout.  Again, the legs are a large muscle group and get strong really fast, so using a much heavier weight is recommended. If you were using a 10lb weight in your first workout, you should be using 20lbs now. Make sure you keep the back straight and bring the dumbbell as close to the floor as possible.

## 6. Side laterals-shoulders (side deltoids)

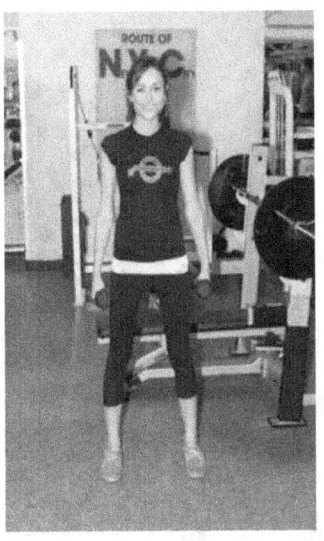
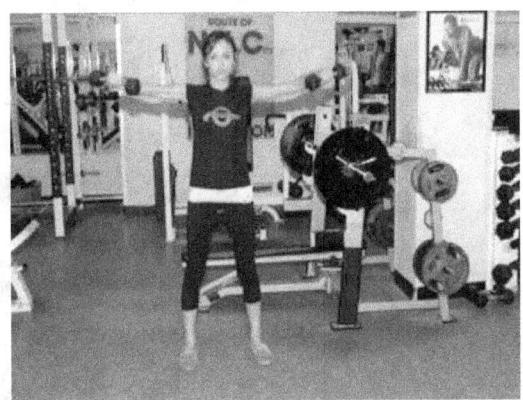

When performing the side lateral you should be focusing on the side deltoid, which is the muscle which gives your shoulders the round look. In men it makes the shoulders appear larger, and it gives women a nice curve on the shoulders.  Start with your hands at your sides, palms facing towards your body.  Use about half the weight you would use on the shoulder press. Raise both arms together, keeping both palms facing toward the floor. Keep the elbow slightly bent at all times.  As you are raising the weight, your hands are turning as if they were pouring a glass of water.  This enables you to keep the elbows slightly higher than the shoulders.  The form is a little tricky at first, but even if it's not perfect you are still working your side deltoids. Do  8 reps.

### 7.  Crunches - feet up (abs)

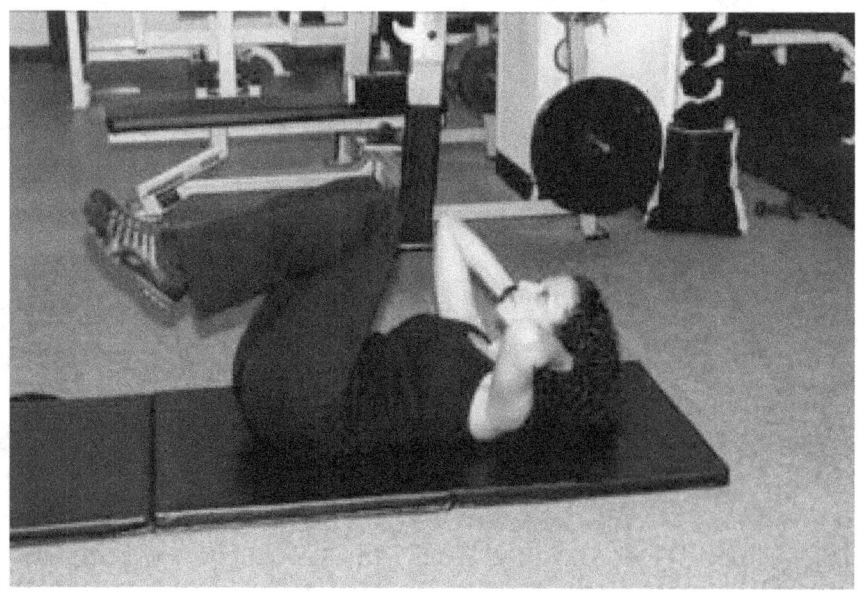

Lay flat with your hands behind your head.  The knees are bent like the regular crunch only you bring our feet off the floor about 18".  As you do your crunch, bring your knees to our elbows, then lower to the starting position. You are only moving your legs about six inches, squeezing the abs and bringing the elbows and knees together at the same time. Try to do slow controlled repetitions starting with 15 and working up to 50 reps.

## 8.  Alternate dumbbell curls-biceps

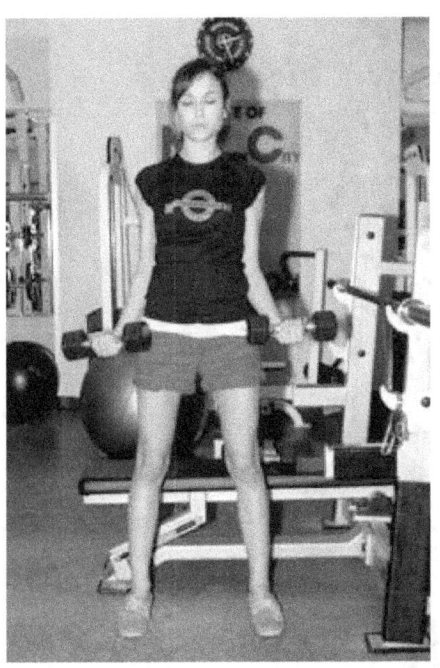 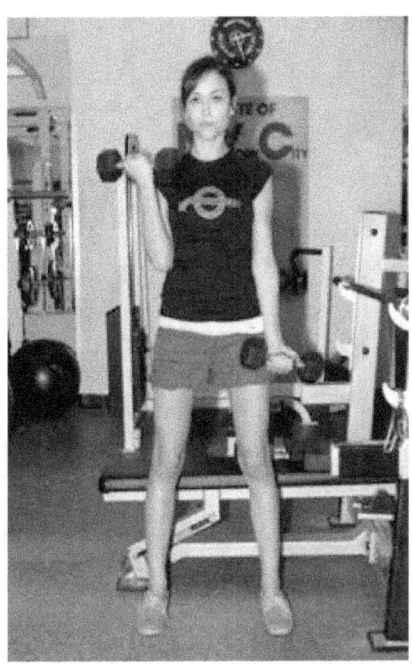

Use the same form as the two arm dumbbell curl, bringing only one arm up at a time.  Start with both arms at your sides and raise your arms until it is about six inches from your shoulder. (see Photo 2). Lower weight and repeat with the other arm. Keep one arm motionless at all times. Do not move both arms at the same time.  Use a weight that is challenging. If you doing 15lbs on your shoulder press, use 10lbs for your curls.

### 9.  Chair dips

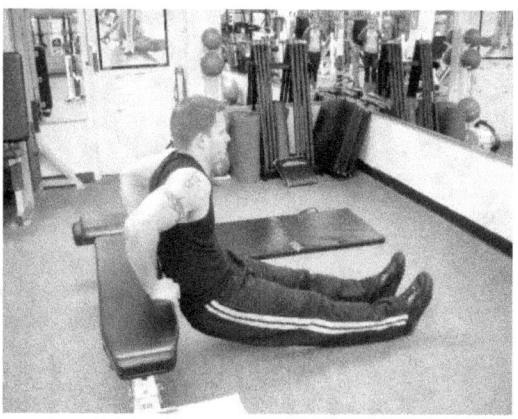

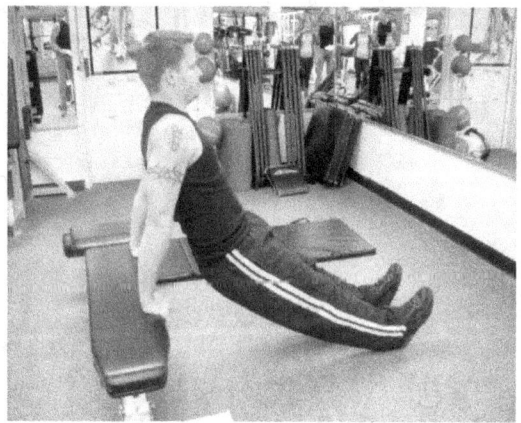

Place both hands behind you on a chair or bench about shoulder width apart.  Extend your legs out in front of the chair. You can make this exercise as hard or easy depending how far you have your legs out in front of you.  If you bend your knees with your feet closer to the chair the easier it is. The farther you have your legs out in front of you, the harder it will be. If your legs are fully extended with your knees locked, the exercise will be the most challenging. Lower your body by bending your elbows; the lower you go, the more effective the exercise will be.

## 10. Bent leg dead lifts- hamstrings, lower back

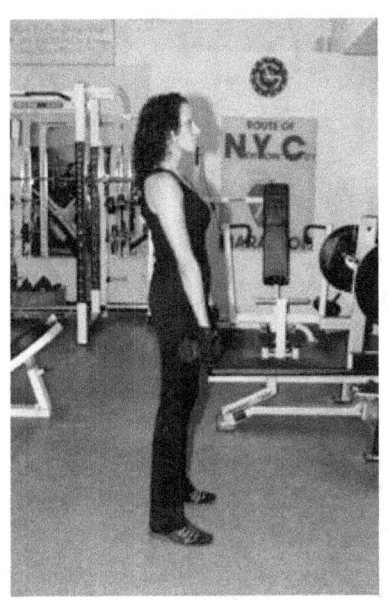 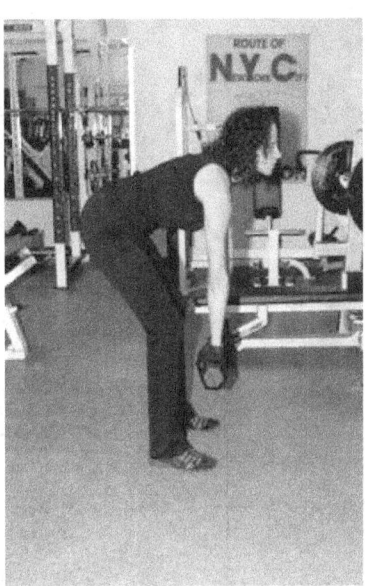

Take a pair of dumbbells about the same weight that you would use for your dumbbell rows. Lower your body, keeping your back arched and your knees slightly bent, arms in front of you (see Photo 2). Raise the weight back to the standing position, (see Photo 1). Lower and repeat. You should feel a good stretch in your lower glutes and hamstrings in the bottom position. Be sure to keep your knees slightly bent at all times. Do 10-15 reps.

## 11. Leg raises- lower abs, quads

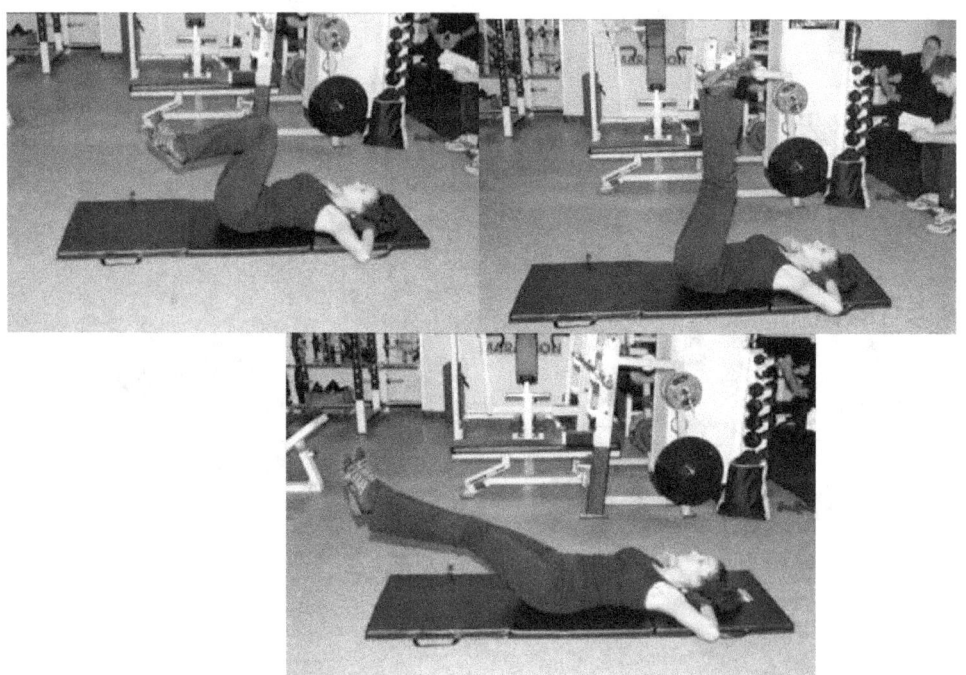

Lie flat on the floor, hands behind your head. Bring your legs up to the position you see in Photo 1 then immediately raise your legs as seen in Photo 2. Lower the legs about 12 inches from the floor as in Photo 3. Do 10-30 reps.

Do this circuit as many times as you like - minimum one, maximum three. Two times would be 20 sets and if you do that in 30 minutes - great job!  One set will probably be enough for now but your goal is two sets by 6 weeks and 3 sets in 10 weeks.

# *16*

## The "B" Workout

You can start your "B" workout whenever you feel you have the ability to do so. The "B" workout isn't necessarily harder, but it has some different exercises and more variety. For example, if you have already been working out before and you can perform a lunge and a squat with proper form then you can do any circuit, A, B, or C.

It is also important in any of these workouts that as we get in better shape we try and use less rest time between exercises as we progress. The goal is very little rest or no rest between each exercise. If you are now using one minute rest between each exercise gradually reduce the time by 5 seconds per exercise per workout. Also make sure you are progressively upping the weights especially in your leg exercises.

### "B" Workout

1. Warm up
2. Lunges
3. Pushups
4. Squats (weight on shoulders)
5. Two-arm dumbbell row
6. Push press
7. Crunches (side to side)
8. Front laterals
9. Triceps kickbacks
10. Leg raises
11. Dumbbell hammer curls
12. Crunches, one leg up alternating legs
13. Plank

**1 .Warm up – Jumping Jacks, Twister swings, Jogging in place**

**2. Lunges – outer thighs, hamstrings, glutes, quadriceps**

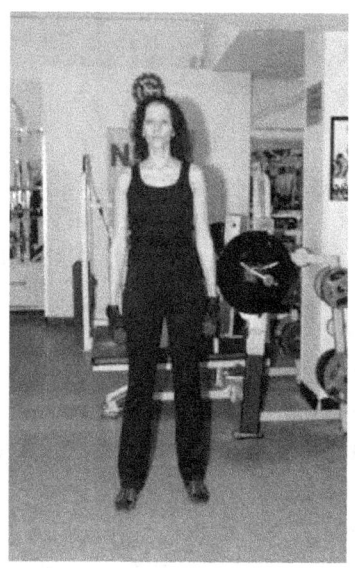 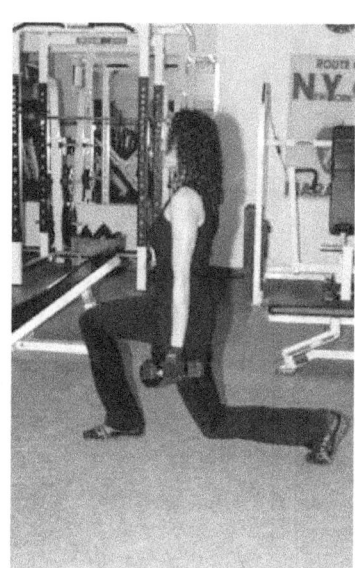

Start with a weight that is lighter than you would use for the squat. You may even want to hold onto a chair for balance if this is your first time doing a lunge.  Have your feet shoulder width apart with the weights hanging by your side, palms facing your body.  See Photo 1. Take a long step forward and lower your body bending your back leg. Your knee should be about six inches from the floor. The better shape you are in the lower you can go. See Photo 2.  As soon as you get into the bottom position, push with the forward leg and come back to the start position. You can alternate legs or use the same leg for five repetitions then switch.  When you get in better shape you can perform ten repetitions with each leg. Tip: your front knee should not extend past your foot.

## 3. Pushups

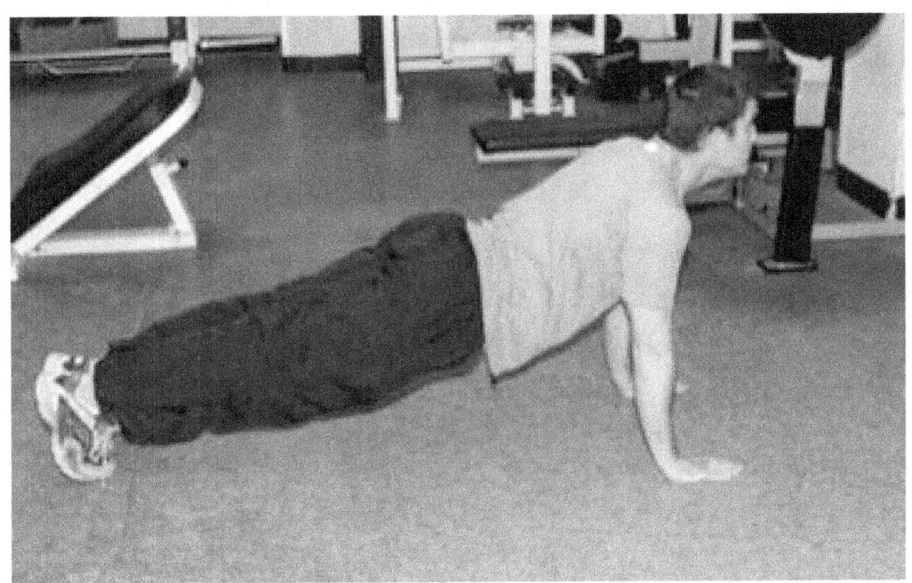

Everyone should know how to do a pushup either from gym class or seeing it done on a fitness video or magazine.  If you can't do a complete pushup stick with the modified pushup from workout A. Start with the position you see the Photo. You may only be able to lower your body six inches and that's ok, but your goal is to lower your body as close to the floor as you can.

## 4. **Squats weight on shoulders**

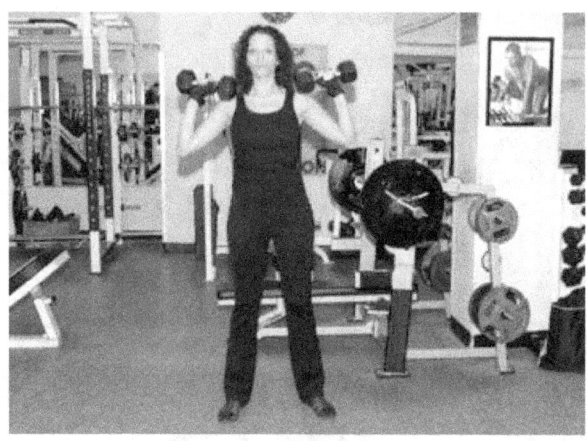

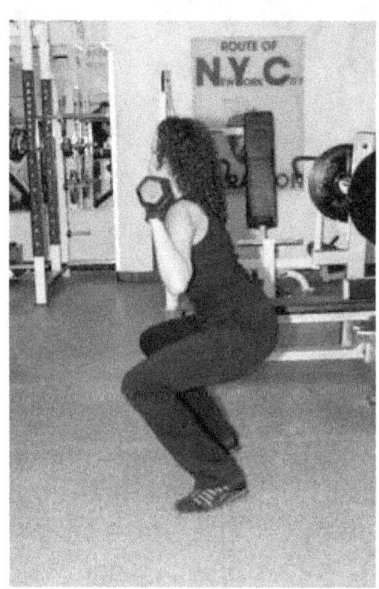

This exercise is similar to the regular squat, except the weight is held on the shoulders. See Photo 1. The front squat enables you to go a little deeper on the squat giving the glutes and thighs a better workout. You can use the same amount of weight you would use on the regular squat, and lower yourself until you get into the position you see in Photo 2.

### 5. Two-arm dumbbell row, back

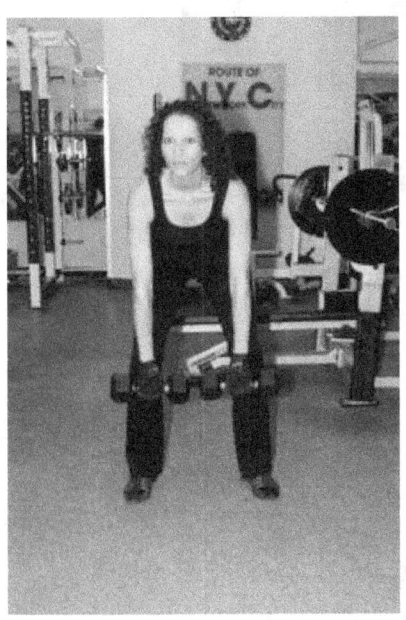 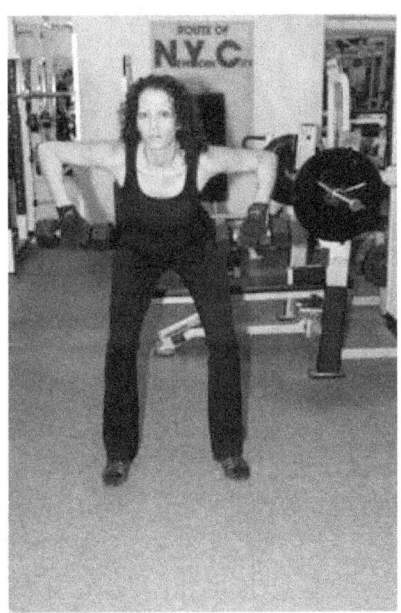

Start in the standing position using fairly heavy dumbbells using the same weight you would use on the squat. Bend forward, keeping your knees slightly bent and back arched at all times. Raise the weights to the position you see in Photo 2. Lower the weights and repeat 10-15 reps. Tip: try to keep your elbows high and bring the weights as close to your chest as possible. At the bottom position be sure to get a good stretch.

## 6. Push press-shoulders, legs

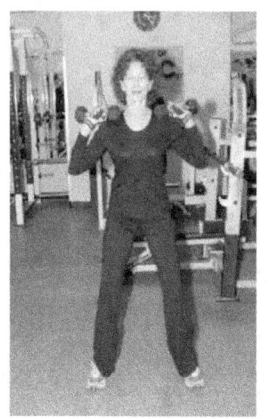 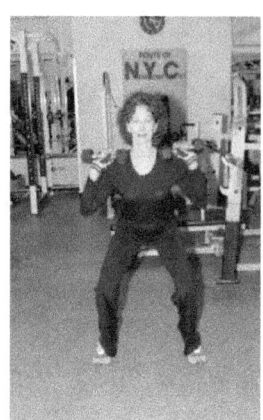

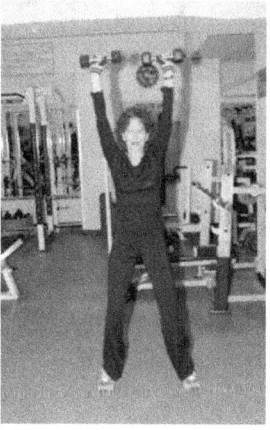

The push press is a good exercise because you are using your arms and legs at the same time.  This makes the exercise more intense and enables you to develop two muscle groups.  Start by using a little heavier weight than you would use on the regular dumbbell press. Remember your legs are doing half of the work.  Start with the dumbbells at your shoulders as you see in Photo 1.  Squat down as low as you can, still holding the weights at your shoulders as you see in Photo 2.  As soon as you get to the bottom part of the squat, press your arms overhead pushing with your legs at the same time.  Your legs and arms should be working together using the same amount of energy. See Photo 3.  Do 8-10 reps.

## 7.  Alternating crunches – side to side 25-50 reps

Get into your regular crunch position with your legs off the floor and knees bent  As you bring your knees to your chest turn your right shoulder to your left knee and then lower.  Turn your left shoulder to your right knee and return to the starting position.

## 8. Front laterals- shoulders, front deltoids

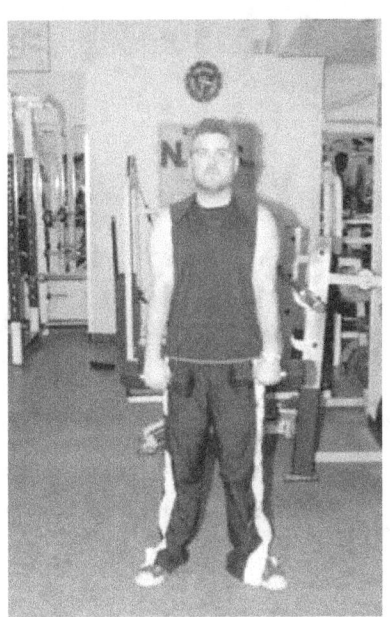
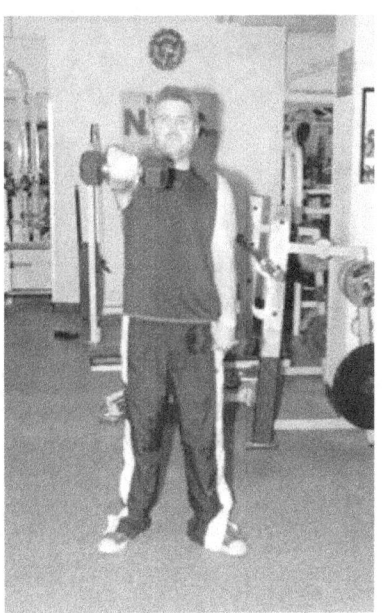

Use a weight that you would use for your side laterals.  Start in the standing position, palms down.  Raise the weight with the elbows slightly bent to shoulder length.  See Photo 2.  Lower and repeat with the other arm.  Always have one arm in the starting position with palms facing the floor.  Remember not to swing the weights. Use a controlled movement, focusing on the muscle group you are working.

## 9. Triceps kickbacks

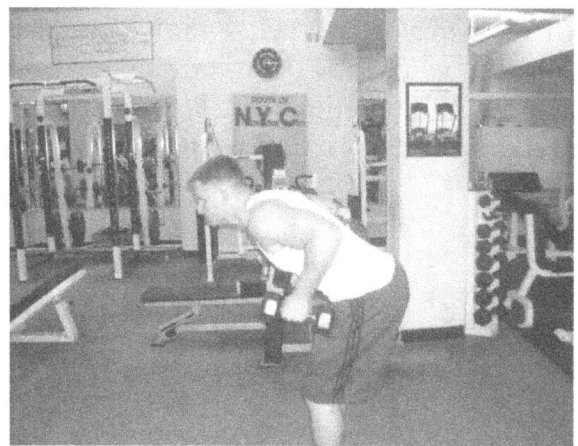

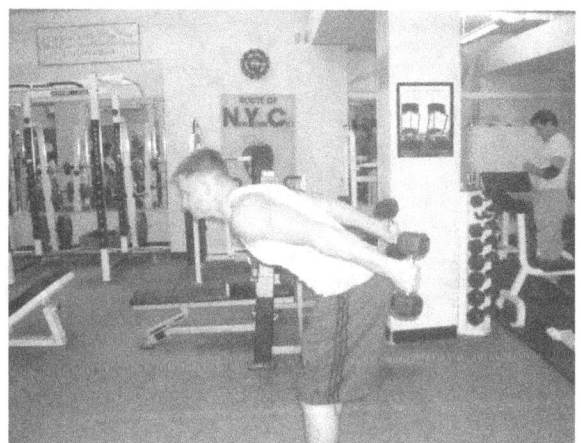

Use a weight that you would use with your front or side laterals. Leaning forward, start with your knees slightly bent with your elbows at your sides, close to your body as seen in Photo 1.  Bring your arms straight back and hold for a split second.  See Photo 2. Try to keep your elbows in the same position at all times while bringing your arms back to the starting position. Do 8-10 reps.

## 10. Leg raises

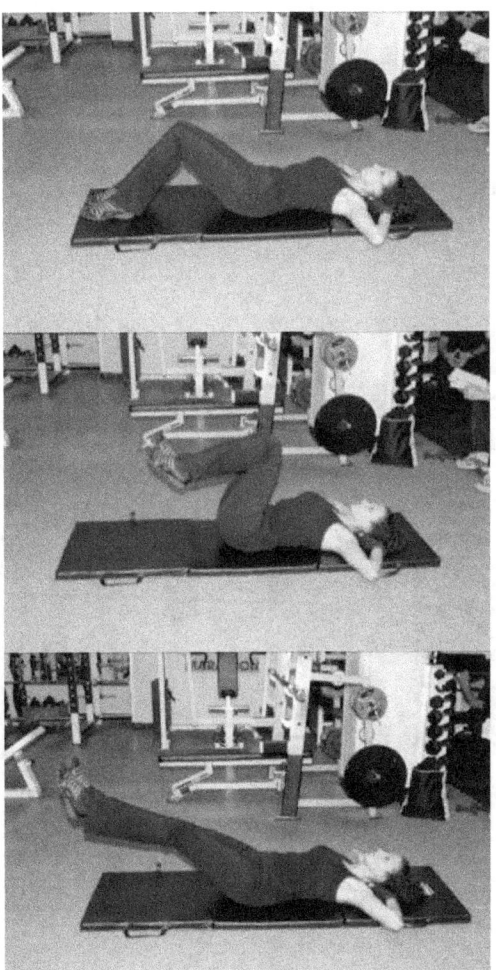

Lie flat on the mat with your legs bent, see Photo 1, bring your knees to your chest, see Photo 2, lower your legs and extend them to the position you see in Photo 3. Keep your feet about 12 inches from the floor. If you feel any pressure on your lower back, put your hands under your glutes, palms down and perform the exercise in the same manner. Do 15-30 reps.

## 11. Dumbbell hammer curls- biceps

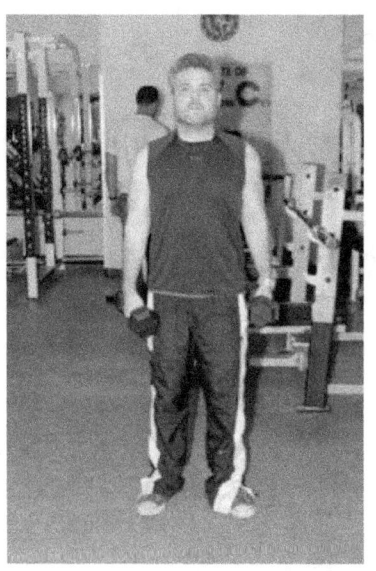 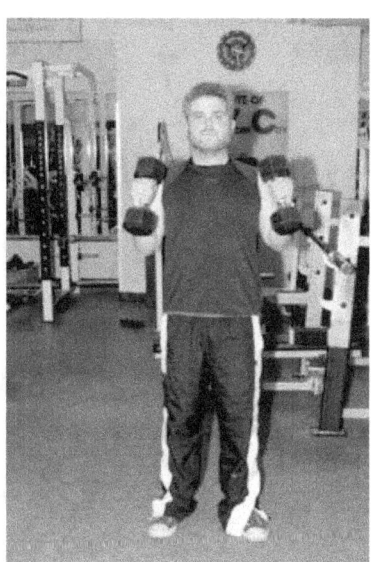

This is a variation of the regular dumbbell curl.  With the weight at your sides, palms facing your body, raise the weight to your shoulders keeping your palms facing each other at all times. See Photo 2. Lower until your arms are completely extended, then repeat.

## 12. Crunches – 1 leg up alternating legs

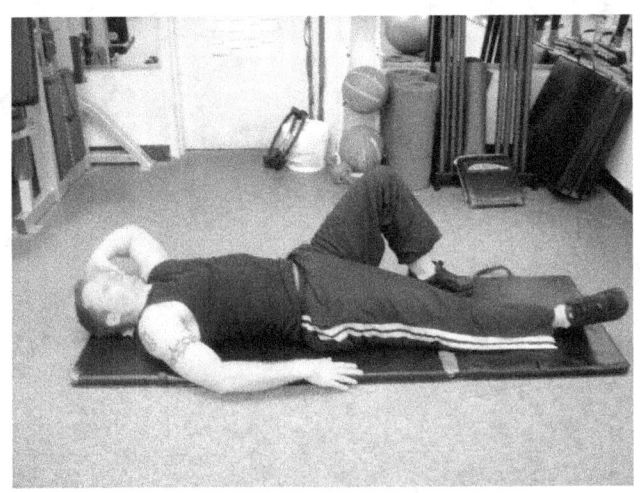

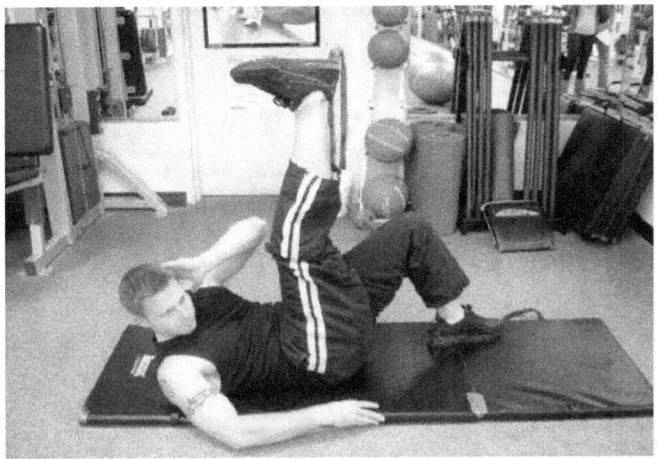

Lie flat on the floor with one leg extended and one leg bent, as shown in Photo 1. Bring the straight leg up to meet the opposite elbow as shown in Photo 2. Lower the leg and repeat. Do 10-15 reps.

### 13. Plank

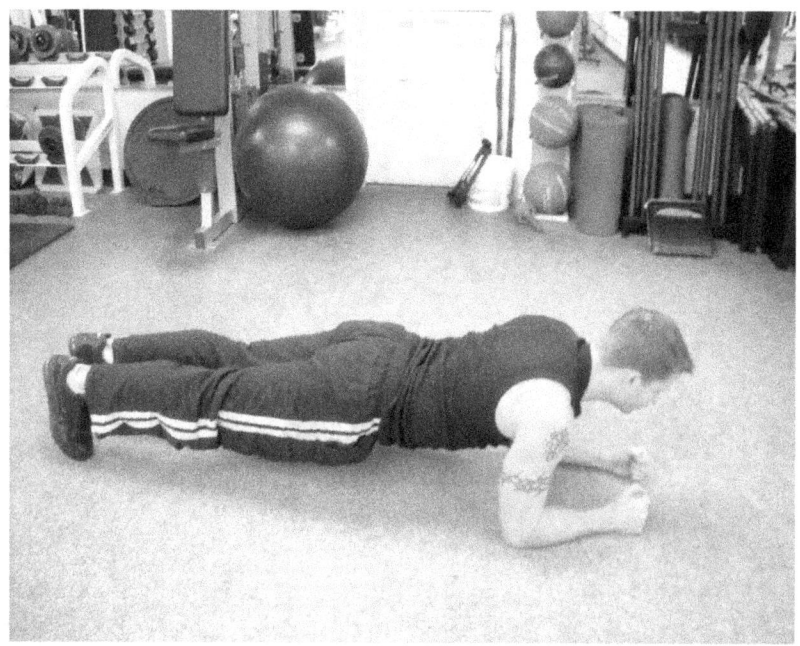

Get into pushup position with your elbows on the floor as seen in the Photo. Hold yourself in that position for 30 seconds, working up to 60 seconds or more. Stabilize with your core to keep your body up in this position.

## Second "B" Routine

The 2nd B routine is similar to the first B routine. You can perform the 1st B routine then go directly into the 2nd for a total of two routines. If you prefer you can do the routines separately but add another set or two and do as many exercises as you like.

I like to put variety into my workout to make things more interesting. Also after a while your body gets used to doing the same exercise and your progress becomes slower. By changing things around your body is challenged differently so it adapts to the stress and progress is made.

Another way to change the intensity of your routine is to switch your workouts around with the order and the amount of repetitions and weight you are doing. For example one day you can perform each exercise for 15 reps with lighter weights and another day you could do heavier weights with fewer repetitions, e.g. 8 reps.

So any routine you do whether it be A, B, or C can be as easy or as hard as you like. Each can take as much time as you like and you will benefit from it. But remember, for optimum results – that is to get a younger body age and a high level of fitness – takes a high intensity 30-minute workout!

## Second"B" Circuit

1. Warm up-10 bodyweight squats, front leg swings

2. 1-arm squat press

3. Close grip pushups

4. Two-arm dumbbell row reverse grip

5. Front side laterals

6. Lunges

7. Side plank

8. Toe Touches

9. Plie' squat weight on shoulders

10. Arnold press

11. Chair dips

12. Crunches legs bent

13. Dumbbell curls

**1.  Warmup – 10 body weight squats, Front leg swings.**

**2.  1-arm squat press**

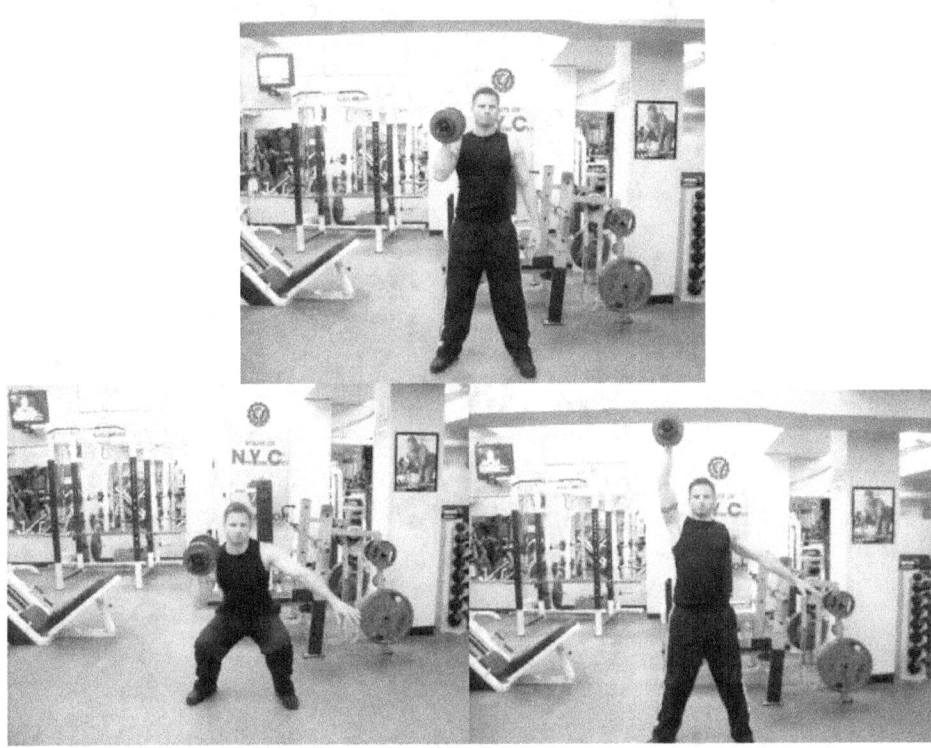

Start out with the dumbbell on your shoulder. Place feet shoulder width apart with abs tight and head up.  Squat down, keeping your weight on your heels.  As you come up, press the dumbbell over your head using your arms and legs at the same time.  Don't go too heavy and sacrifice good form. 8 reps, each arm.

### 3. Close grip pushups

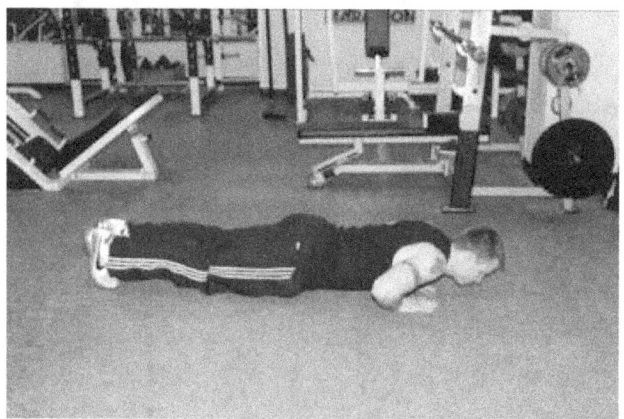

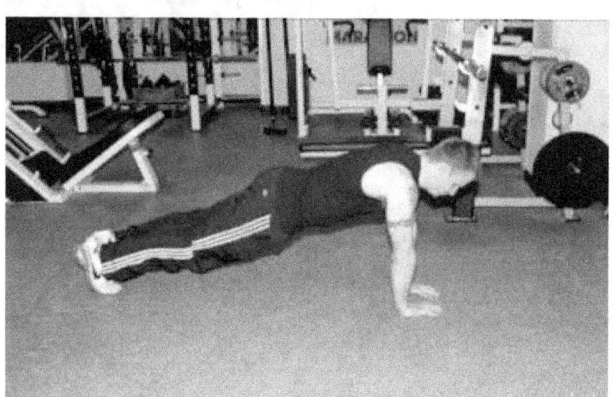

Get into pushup position with hands six inches apart. This is similar to the regular pushup but placing more emphasis on your triceps and working the chest and shoulders as well. If the movement is too difficult at first perform the exercise with your hands on a bench or chair. Try to perform as many repetitions as you can while using good form.

## 4. Two arm dumbbell row with reverse grip

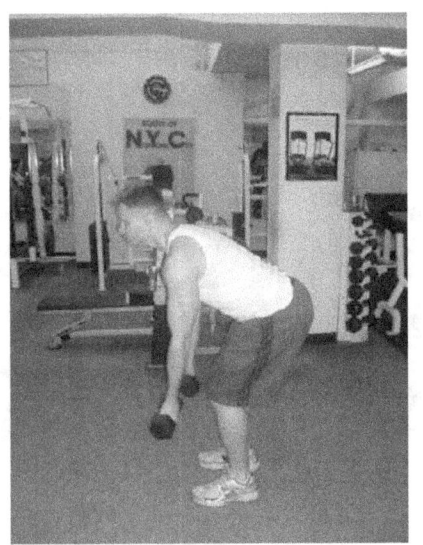 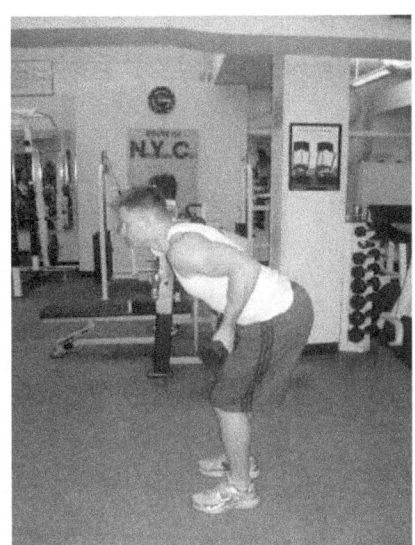

Use the same form you would use on the regular two-arm dumbbell row, only have your palms facing away from you. Bend your knees slightly with your back arched and body leaning forward (see Photo 1). Bring the weights to your chest (see Photo 2) and lower the weights. Repeat. Do 8-10 reps.

## 5. Front side laterals

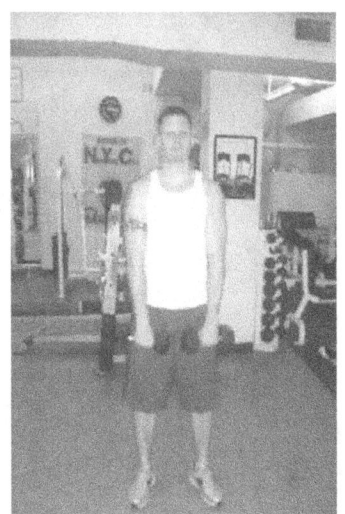
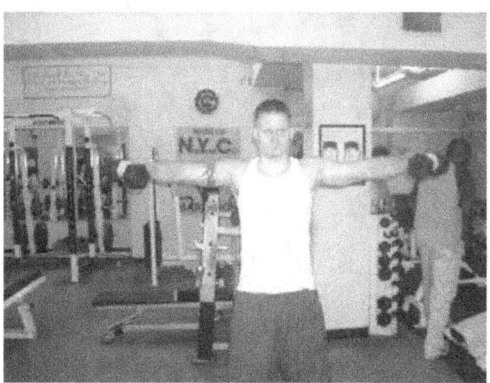

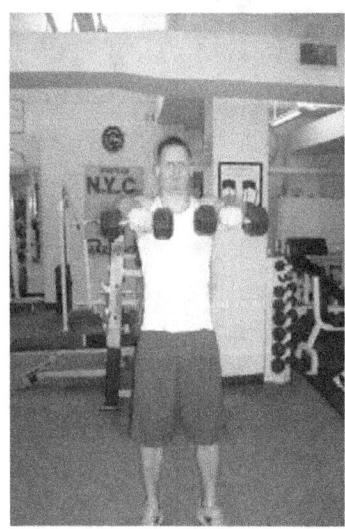

Use the same weight and form you would use on your front and side laterals.  With palms facing in, perform a side lateral, bringing the weight down to your sides then immediately perform a front lateral. Perform five repetitions with the front lateral and five with the side lateral. The exercise can be done with one arm at a time or with both arms together.

## 6.  Lunges, weights at your side

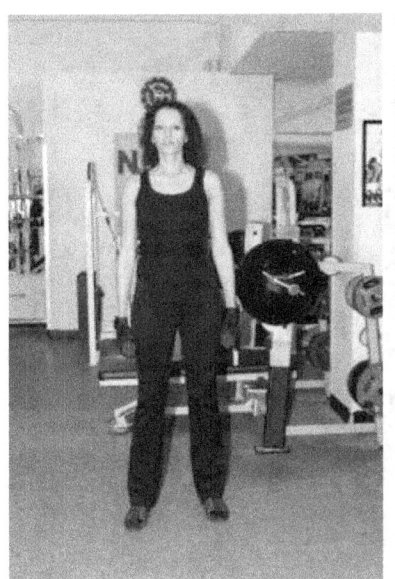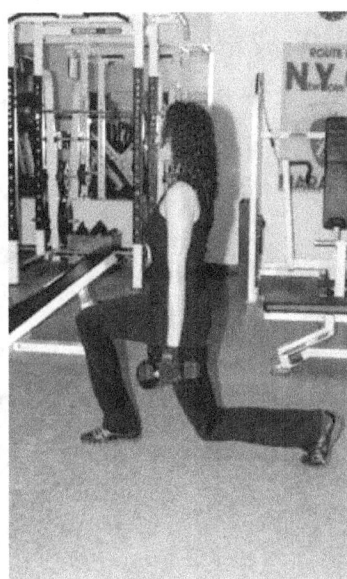

Use the same form you did on your B workout but try and use a heavier weight.  Do 10-15 reps.

## 7.  Side Plank

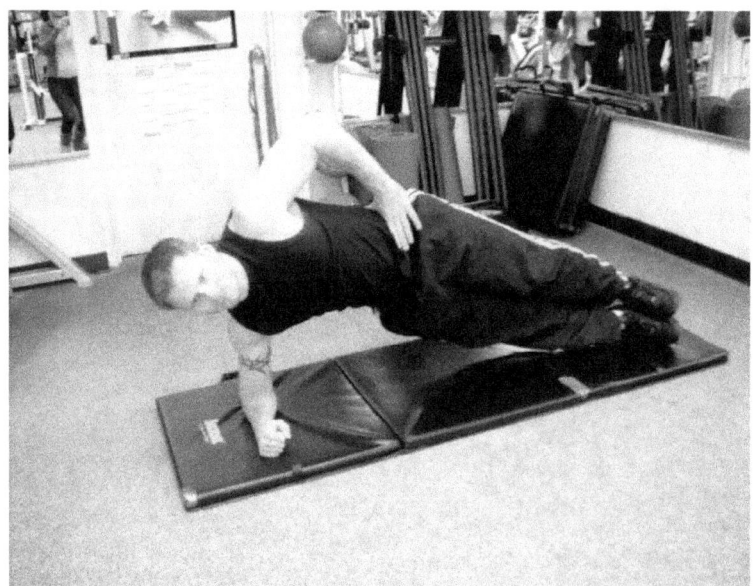

This is similar to the regular plank only you are on your side with bodyweight on one elbow.  Make sure you stabilize your body with your core.   Hold the position for 30-60 seconds then change sides. This exercise works your core with the emphasis on your obliques.

## 8. Toe Touches

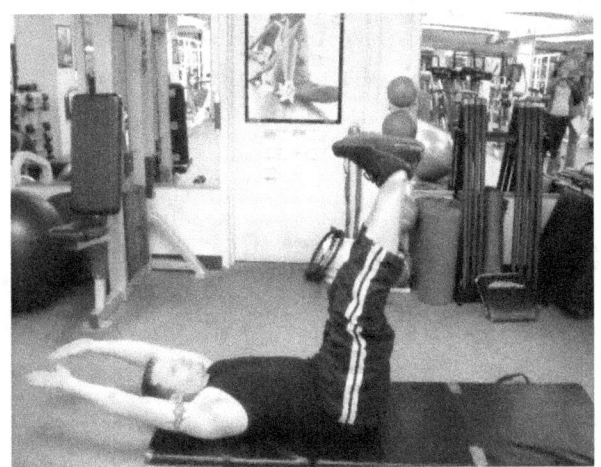

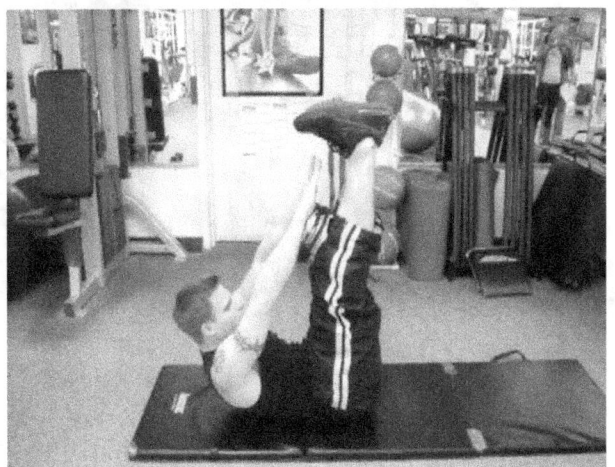

Lying on your back with feet straight up, crunch up as high as you can as if you were touching your toes. Go back to the starting position and repeat 10-20 times. Tip: As you bring your upper body toward your toes, try to squeeze your abs at all times.

## 9.  Plie' squat weight on shoulder- inner thighs, glutes

This exercise is similar to the regular plie' squat only the weights are held on your shoulders making it more difficult to do.  Use the same amount of weight you would use on your regular squat.  Put your legs about two feet apart, keeping the feet in the plie position. Keeping your back straight, squat as low as you can.  You should be in good enough shape by now to go very deep on your squat, putting emphasis on your inner thighs.  10-15 reps

## 10. Arnold press – shoulders and biceps

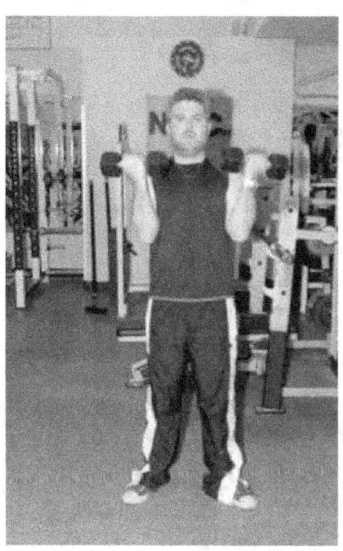 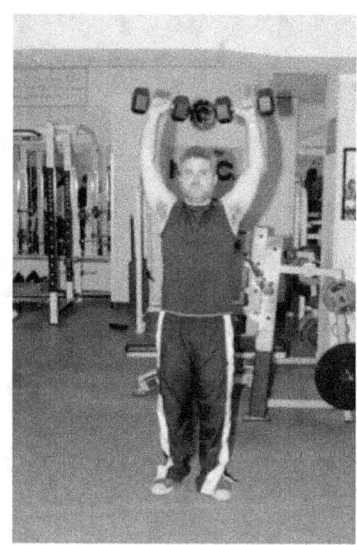

This is a variation of the regular press but was developed by Arnold Schwarzenegger. It gives the press a fuller range of motion and incorporates the biceps into the exercise. Start with two dumbbells with the same weight you would use in the regular dumbbell press only have your palms facing the body instead of away from the body. See Photo 1. As you press the weight overhead, turn your wrists so at the top of the movement your palms are facing away from the body. See Photo 2.  While lowering the weight, turn your palms in the opposite direction so that when your palms reach your shoulder, they are facing your body.  Do 8-10 reps.

## 11. Chair dips

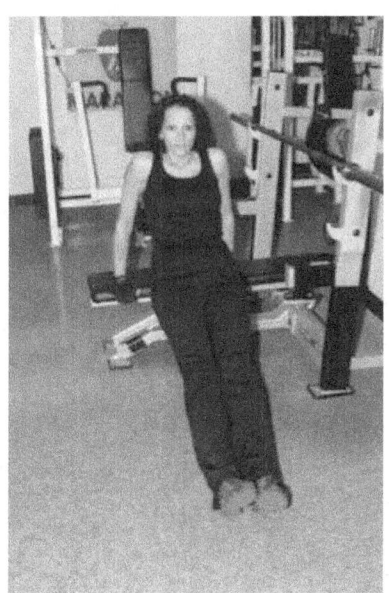 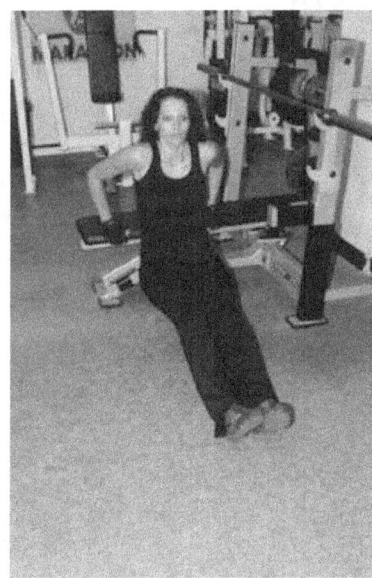

Use the same form as the second A workout. You should be able to move your feet farther away from your body to make it more difficult. When your legs are extended straight out with your knees in a locked position, your triceps are worked the hardest. Also the lower you go, the harder the exercise becomes. Do 15-20 reps

### 12. Crunches – legs bent bring knees to chest

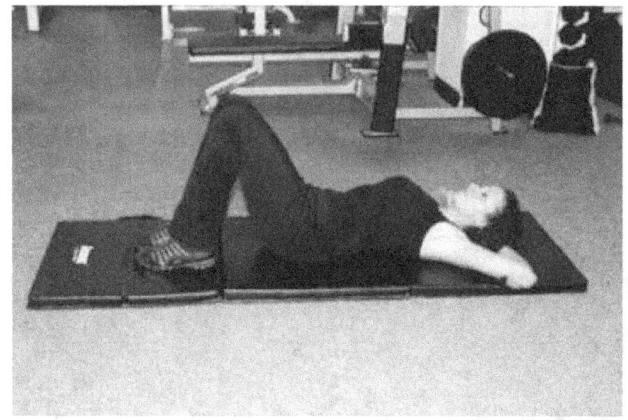

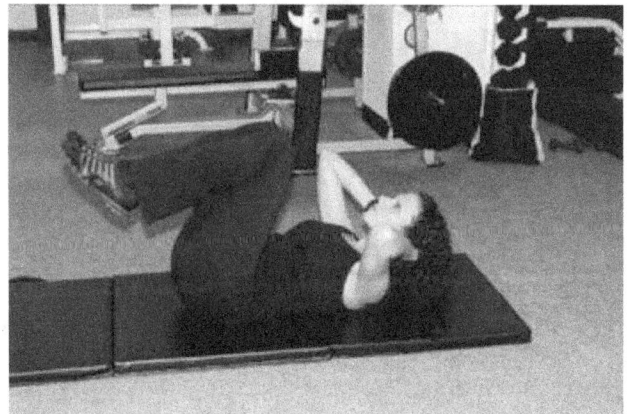

Start in the lying down crunch position.  Bring your knees straight up as shown in Photo 2.  As you raise our head to perform a crunch,  bring in the knees to your elbows and lower to the start position.  Perform slow and controlled movements, trying to keep your abs tight at all times. The total distance that you bring our knees towards your elbows should be no longer than 12 inches.  Do 30-50 reps.

### 13. Dumbbell curl

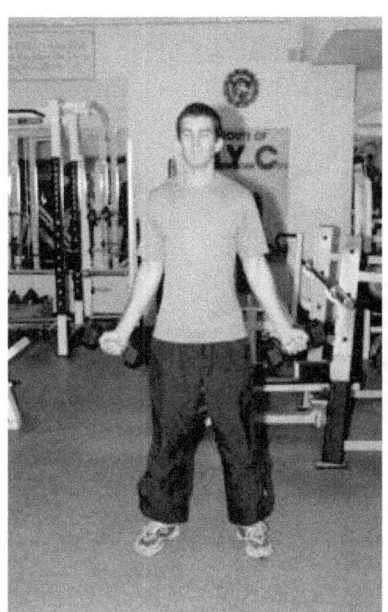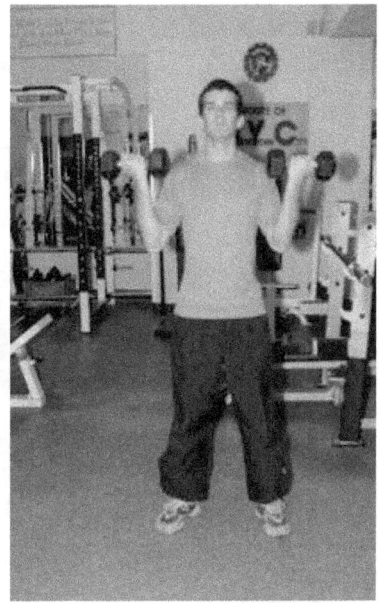

Use the same form as the first A workout. You should also be using a lot more weight than when you first started.  When you perform a curl you should not bring the weight all the way to your shoulders, stop about six inches before you reach them. Do 8-10 reps

I'm a lawyer so I don't have time to spend an hour in the gym. Since I've been working out using the 30 minute workouts with Art, I'm twice as strong as I used to be and my tennis has improved dramatically!

...Jeff Hoffman, 66

# *17*

## The "C" Routine

Your level C workout will add some more variety and some new challenges to your routines.  Again you don't have to add these routines to get results but if you want to take your workouts a bit farther, then this is for you. You will need a little more equipment to do them, either a flat bench or a stability ball.  A stability ball can be purchased in any sports store and takes up very little room in your house. A flat bench is a bit more expensive but it is a good piece of equipment to have. Either one will do just fine in your workout.  In the level C workout I will list a good number of exercises. You can do them with little rest and go straight through without stopping or you can use heavier weights and take more rest. Do about 8 repetitions on the upper body exercises and 10 on the leg exercises. Do between 20 and 50 reps on your crunches and as many pushups as you can do. Two circuits of the following would be a good workout in 30 minutes.

1.  Pushups
2.  Flat bench dumbbell press
3.  Flat bench dumbbell fly
4.  Split Squat
5.  Alternating  dumbbell press
6.  Lunge with side laterals
7.  Reverse Flies
8.  Roll ups on Ball
9.  Pullovers
10.  Stability ball crunch
11. Lunges with Dumbbell curls
12. Upright rows
13. Jackknife
14. Lying triceps extension
15. Plank on Ball

**1. Pushups 25-35**

**2. Flat bench dumbbell press – chest, shoulders, triceps 2 sets, 1st set warm up**

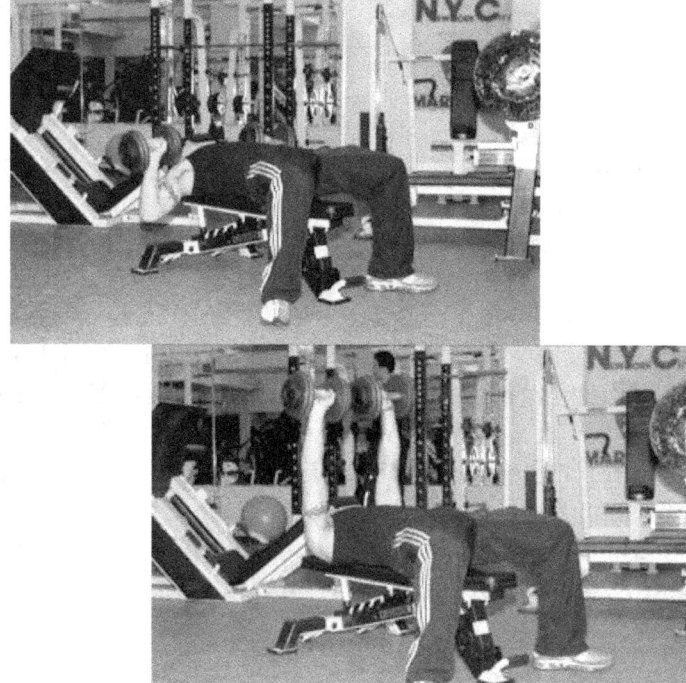

Start with a pair of dumbbells that are heavier than you would use on your shoulder press. Holding the weights about shoulder width apart, press the weights straight up as shown in the Photo 2. Use the first set as a warm up, and use a heavier weight on your second set. It may take a few times doing this exercise to get used to controlling the weight. When you start your press from the bottom position, you should press straight up and bring the weights closer to each other on the finishing position. When lowering the weight bring the weights wider to get to the shoulder width position at the bottom.

### 3.  Flat dumbbell flies, 2 sets

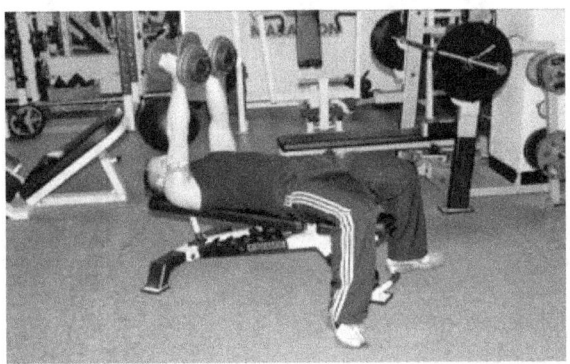

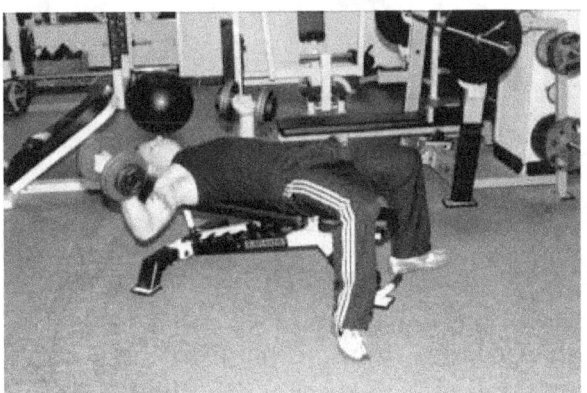

Start with a lighter weight than you would use with the dumbbell bench press.  See Photo 1.  With your arms directly overhead and palms facing each other, lower the weight slowly with a four-second count to the position used in Photo 2.  You should feel a nice stretch in your chest at the bottom movement.  Keep your elbows bent at all times on the bottom position. Raise the weights like you were hugging a large tree and end at the starting position. Remember to control the weight on the way down while feeling a good stretch and then bring the weights to the top position.  Do 8-10 reps.

### 4. Split Squats

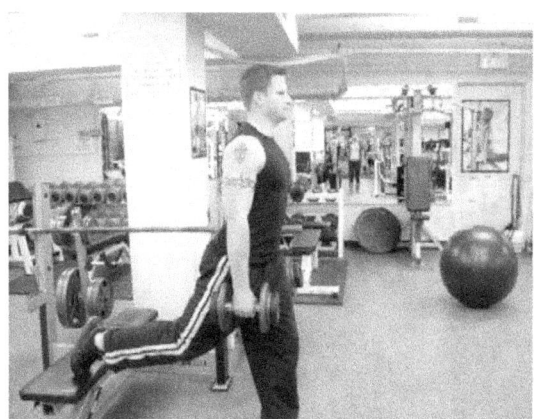 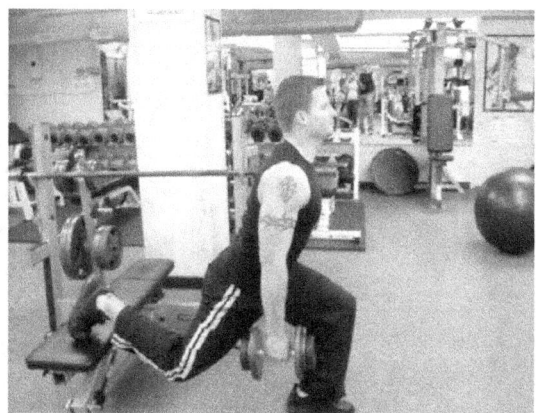

Stand about three feet in front of a bench or chair and place your back leg on the bench, touching it with your toes. Keep your stance wide enough that your knee stays behind your toes when you lunge down. Squat with your front leg, bending both knees into a lunge position. Maintaining your balance, push back to the starting position.  Perform 10 reps then switch legs.  Add weight when necessary.

## 5. Alternate dumbbell press.

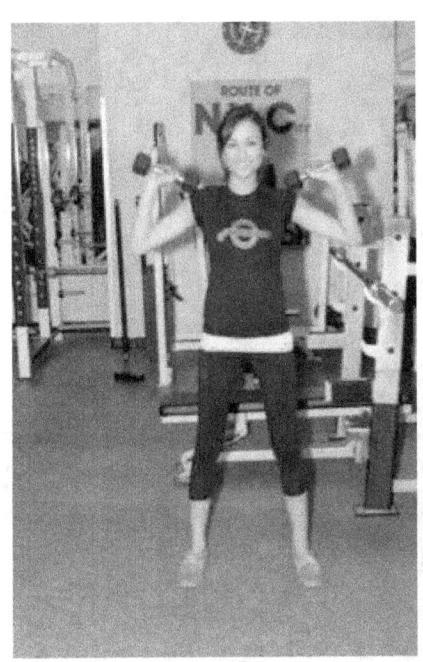 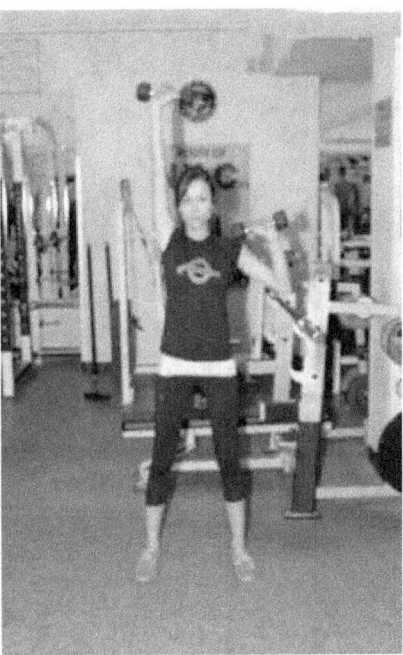

Perform the exercise the same way you would do a two-arm dumbbell press but only use one arm at a time. See Photo 1. Do 8-10 reps. Tip: make sure you keep one weight on the shoulder at all times as your other arm goes straight up.

### 6. Lunge with side laterals.

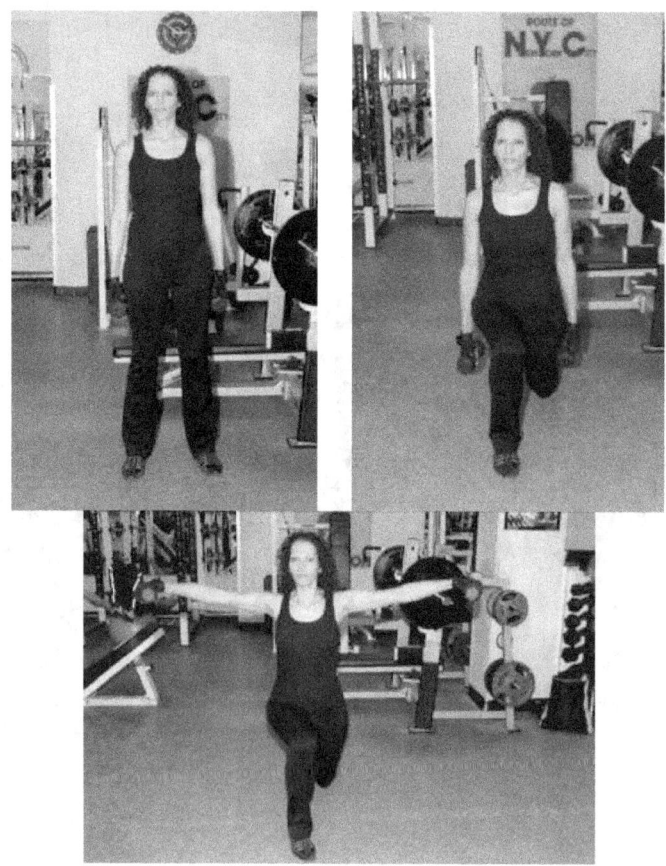

This is a great exercise combining the upper and lower body. Use a weight you would normally use for a side lateral. You already know how to do a lunge and a side lateral, all we are doing is combining the two. As you drop in the bottom lunge position hold the position and perform a side lateral. See Photo 3. After you complete the lateral, immediately return to the starting position and switch legs. Perform five reps per leg with a total of 10 repetitions with the lunge and 10 with the side lateral.

## 7.  Reverse Flies

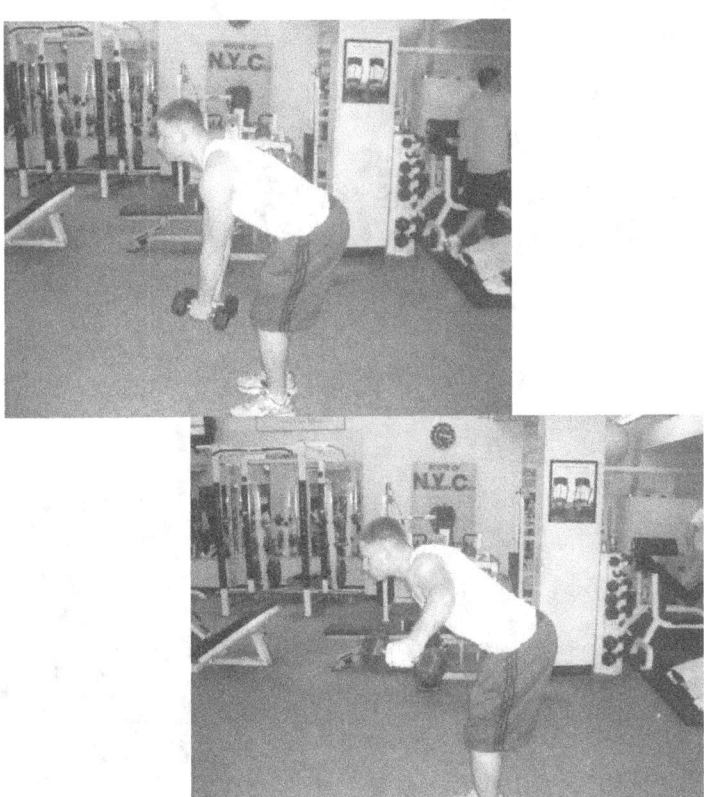

This is a great rear deltoid exercise. Bend over with the knees slightly bent and back arched. Keeping the elbows slightly bent, do a side lateral, squeezing the shoulders blades to focus on the rear delts.  Use the same weight you would use doing a side lateral. Do 8-10 reps

## 8.  Roll ups on Ball (Core)

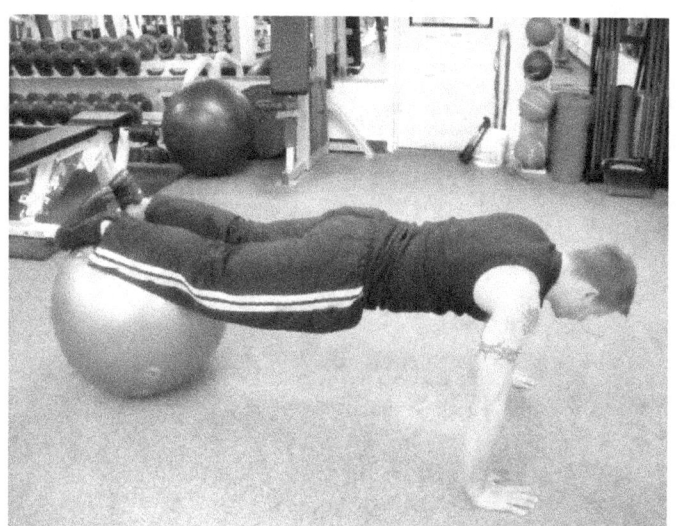

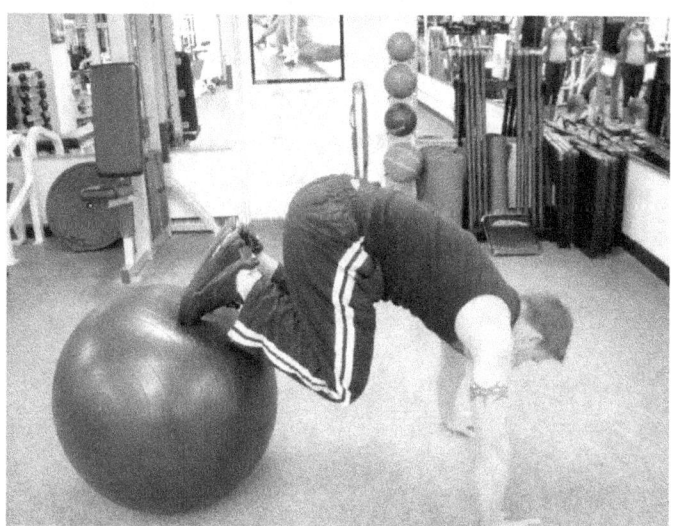

Get into pushup position with feet on the ball shown in Photo 1. Slowly bend your knees, bringing the ball toward your body as close to your chest as possible. Return the ball back to starting position and repeat 10-15 times.

### 9. Pullovers (chest, back, triceps)

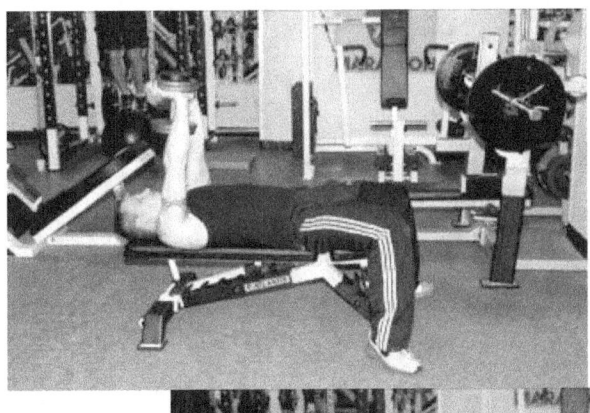

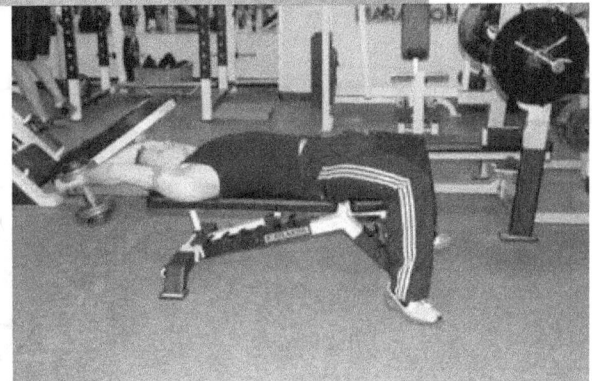

The pullover is a great exercise because it incorporates more than one muscle group. It also stretches the muscles while strengthening them at the same time. Use about the same weight you would use on your shoulder press. Lie flat on a bench, holding the dumbbell at the top with your palms facing toward the ceiling. See Photo 1. Slowly lower the weight keeping your elbows slightly bent until you get to the position shown in Photo 2. You should feel a good stretch when you get to the bottom of the movement, going as low as you can with the dumbbell. Return to the starting position and repeat.

### 10. Stability ball crunch

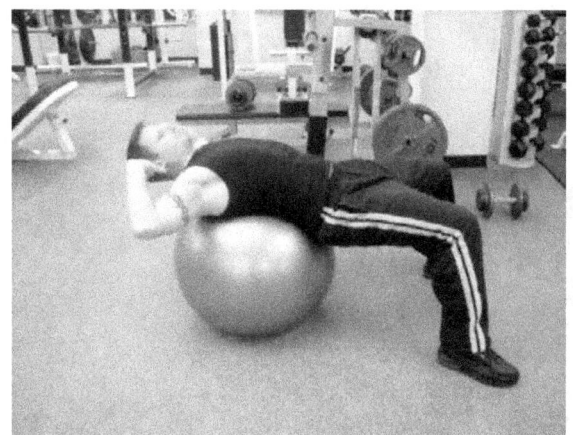

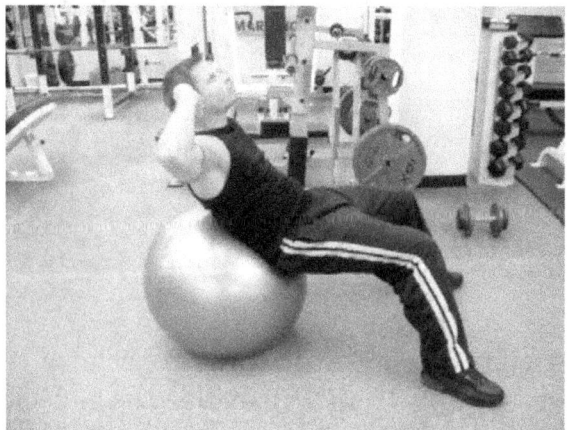

Lie on a stability ball with your head behind the ball as seen in Photo 1. Using your abs, crunch up to the position you see in Photo 2. Do 25 – 50 reps.

### 11. Lunges with dumbbell curl (legs, biceps)

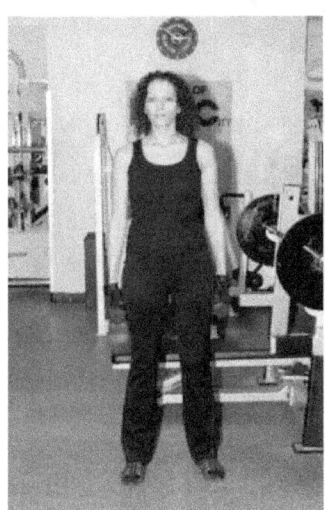 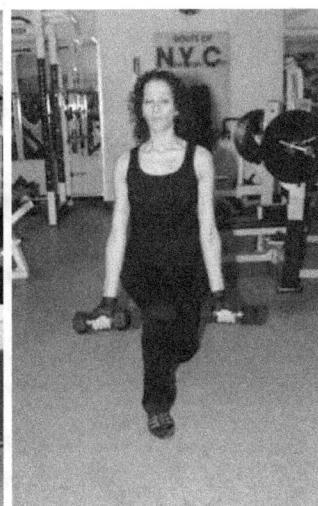 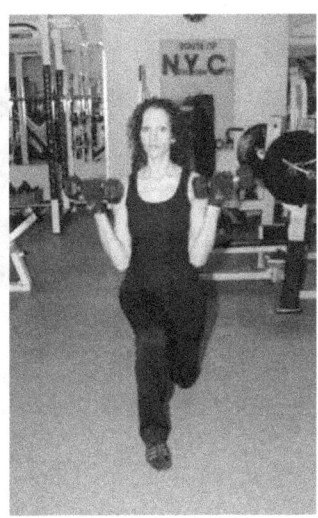

Starting in a standing position, palms facing your sides, drop into the bottom lunge position, hold the position as seen in Photo 2, and perform a dumbbell curl as in Photo 3. After you complete the curl, immediately return to the starting position and switch legs. Perform 5 reps with each leg on the lunge with a total of 10 lunges and 10 curls.

## 12. Upright rows (shoulders, traps)

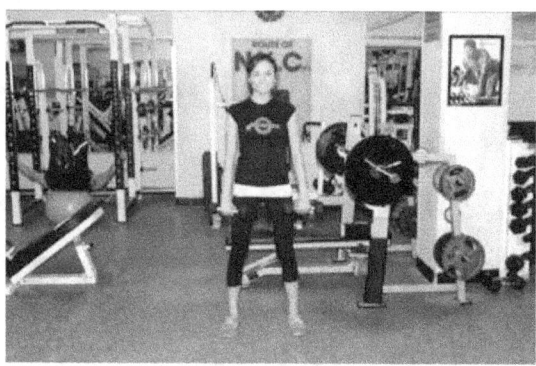

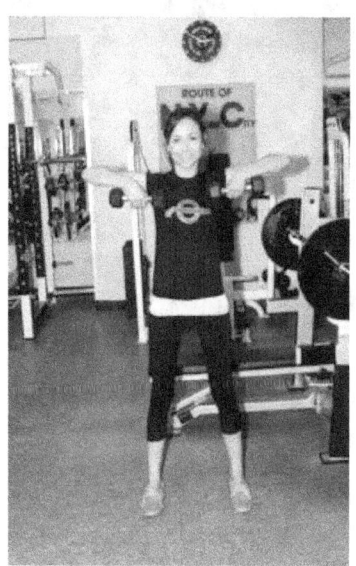

Start in the standing position, palms facing the body.  Use a pair of dumbbells you would normally use for your shoulder press. Keep the arms close to your body, keeping the dumbbell about 12 inches apart. See Photo 1. Raise the arms to shoulder level.  An important part of the exercise is to keep the elbows up as seen in Photo 2.  Lower and repeat, 8-10 times.

## 13. Jackknife (abs)

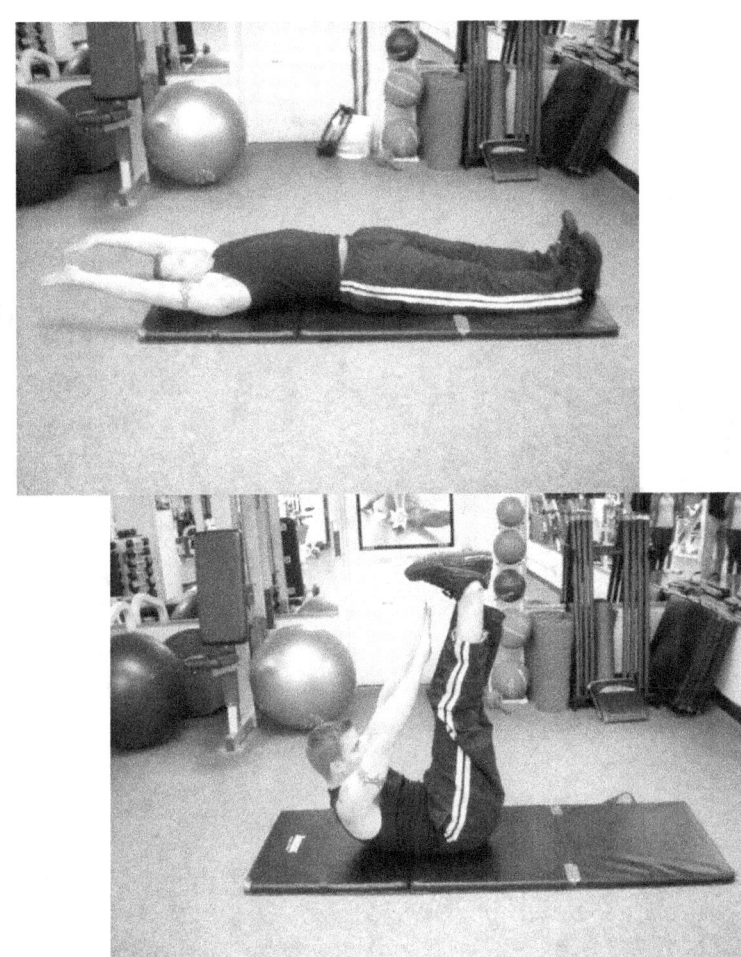

This is an advanced exercise that works both lower and upper abs. Lie flat with arms extended over head, see Photo 1. Raise arms and legs at the same time until they meet as in Photo 2, then return to the starting position. At first it will be hard to keep your balance, but as you get used to the exercise it will become easier. When you get better at the movement you can hold the top position for 1-3 seconds.

## 14. Lying tricep extension

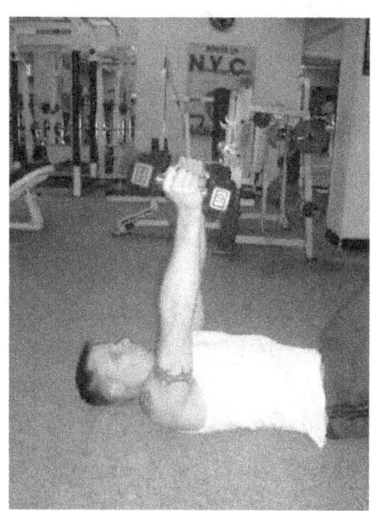
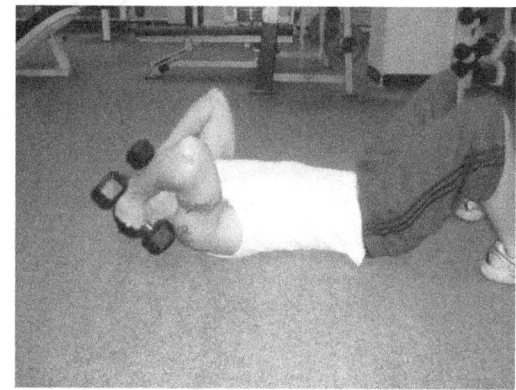

Use a dumbbell that is heavy enough that you could only perform 10 reps. Lie flat on a bench or floor, arms extended straight up with palms facing each other. See Photo 1.  Keeping your elbows back toward your body,  lower both dumbbells to your shoulders. See Photo 2. Then raise to starting position.

### 15. Plank on Ball

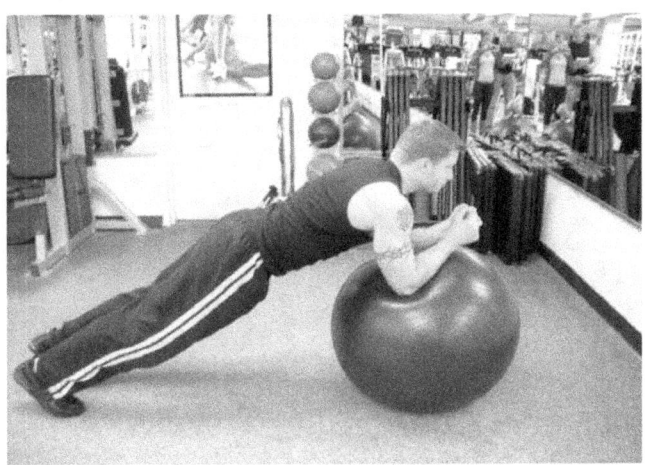

This is an advanced version of the plank. The Plank is a great exercise for endurance in your abs and back as well as for stabilization.  On a ball, start by lying face down. Get into pushup position with elbows and forearms on the ball. See Photo. Keep your back flat and in a straight line, contract your abs and hold the position for 20-60 seconds. The farther the ball is in front of you, the harder it becomes.

I have given you a lot of exercises to practice. You can do the whole routine as is or you can develop your own routine and use some of the exercises.  You will have to be in fairly good shape to perform some of the movements at level C. Your goal again is a 30-minute workout doing as many exercises as you can. In the second C workout I'm going to add some exercises we haven't done before that you can incorporate in any of your other routines.

## Second "C" Workout

1. Flat press on stability ball

2. Dumbbell Flies on ball

3. Split squat on ball

4. Roll ups on ball straight leg

5. Push up on ball

6. Jump Squat

7. Romanian Twist

8. Squat Arnold Press

9. Pullovers on ball

10. Triceps extension on ball

11. Stability Ball Crunch with dumbbell

12. Walking Lunges

13. Plank Pushups

14. Reverse fly on ball

15. Concentration Curl

## 1. Flat press on stability ball

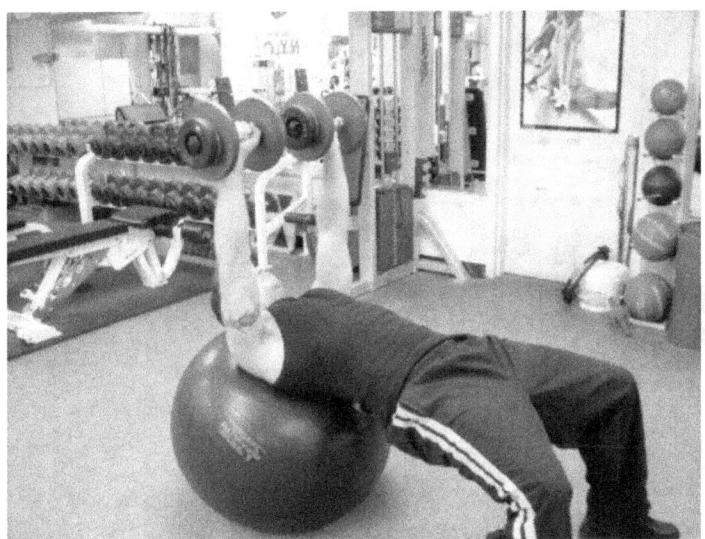

Lie flat on a stability ball as shown in the Photo.  Use the same form you would use on a flat bench dumbbell press. It will be hard to maintain your balance at first so start by using a lighter weight than usual.

## 2. Dumbbell flies on ball

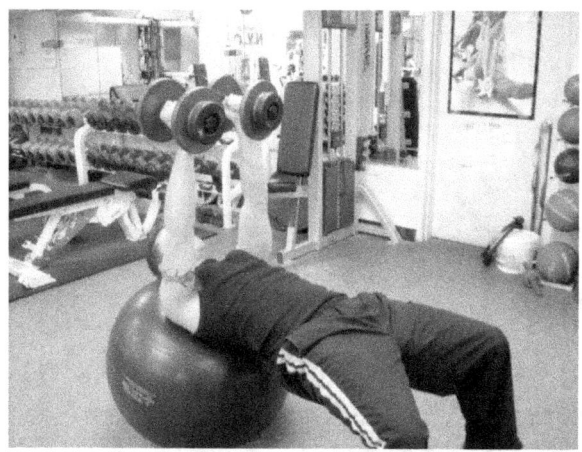

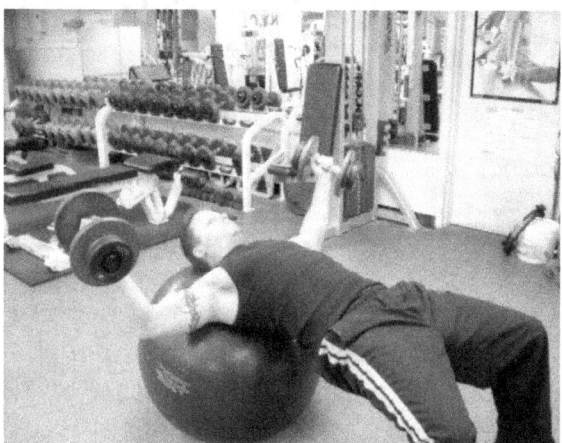

Use the same form you would on a flat bench dumbbell fly, only perform the exercise on a stability ball.

### 3. Split Squat on ball

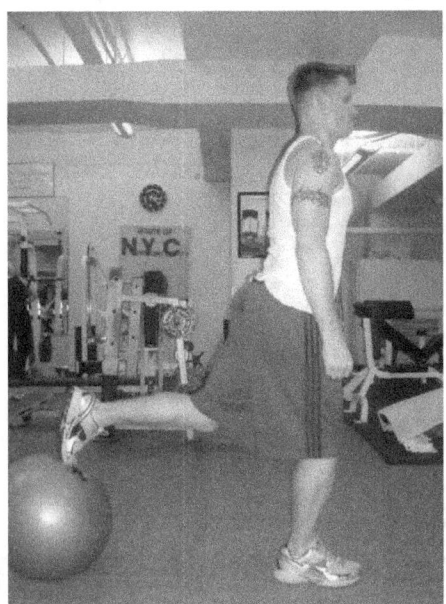 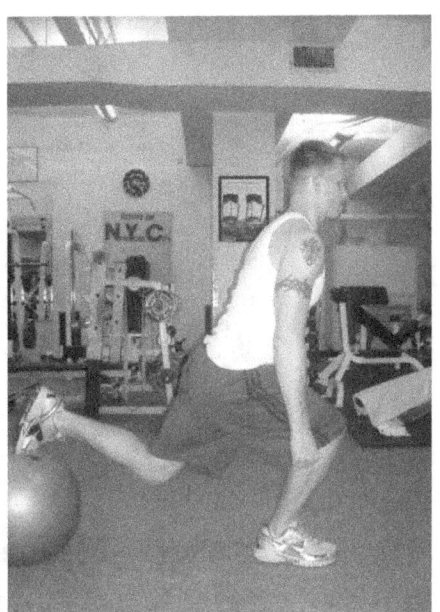

This is an advanced exercise that requires a lot of balance as well as strength to perform. Use the same form you would use on the split squat on a bench or chair.  Start with no weights until you balance improves. Do 10 reps.

### 4. Roll ups on ball straight leg

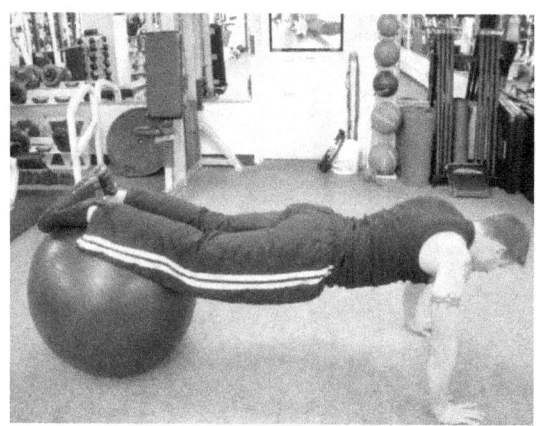

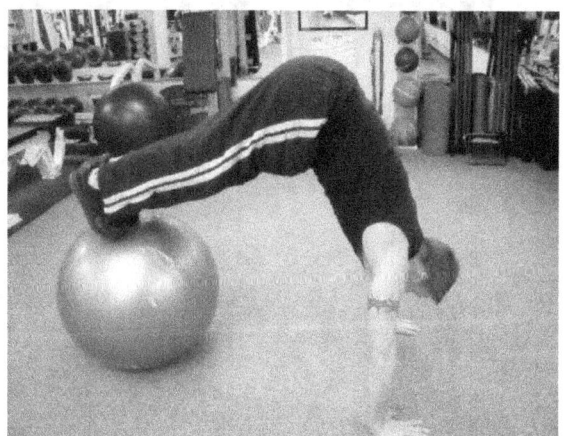

Get into pushup position on a stability ball. Instead of bending your knees and rolling the ball up with your legs bent, keep your legs straight, knees locked, as seen in Photo 2 and bring the ball as close to your upper body as you can. Lower and repeat 10-20 repetitions.

### 5.  Pushup on ball

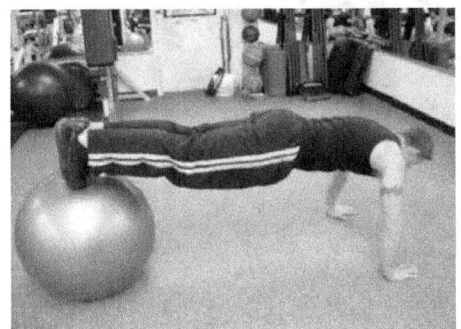

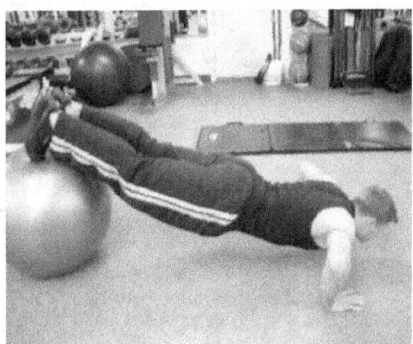

Do a regular pushup with your feet on the stability ball behind you. Perform as many repetitions as you can.

### 6.  Jump Squat

This is an advanced plyometric move that develops power in the legs. Athletes use this exercise to increase their speed and jumping ability as well their strength and flexibility in the legs. With two dumbbells at your side, squat down to a parallel position and immediately jump straight up, trying to bring your knees to your chest.  You can also try to jump squat with no weights at first. Perform 10 reps.

### 7.  Romanian Twist

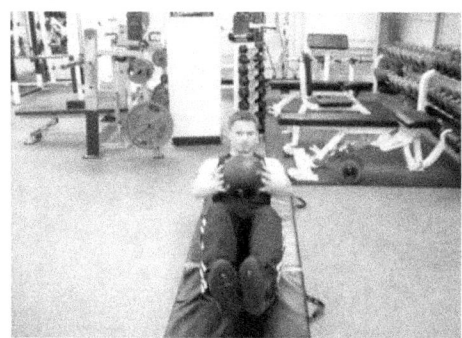

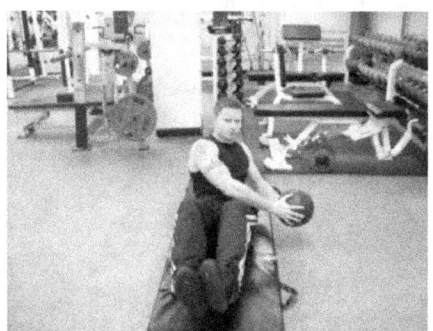

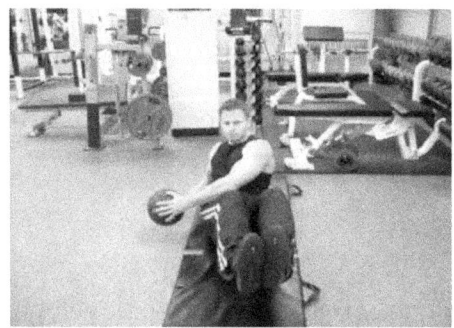

Sit down on the floor and lean back until your abs engage. Lift up your feet approximately six inches from the floor. With a medicine ball or weight, twist from side to side. Use a light weight at first. Do 15 reps then increase to 25.

### 8.  Squat Arnold Press

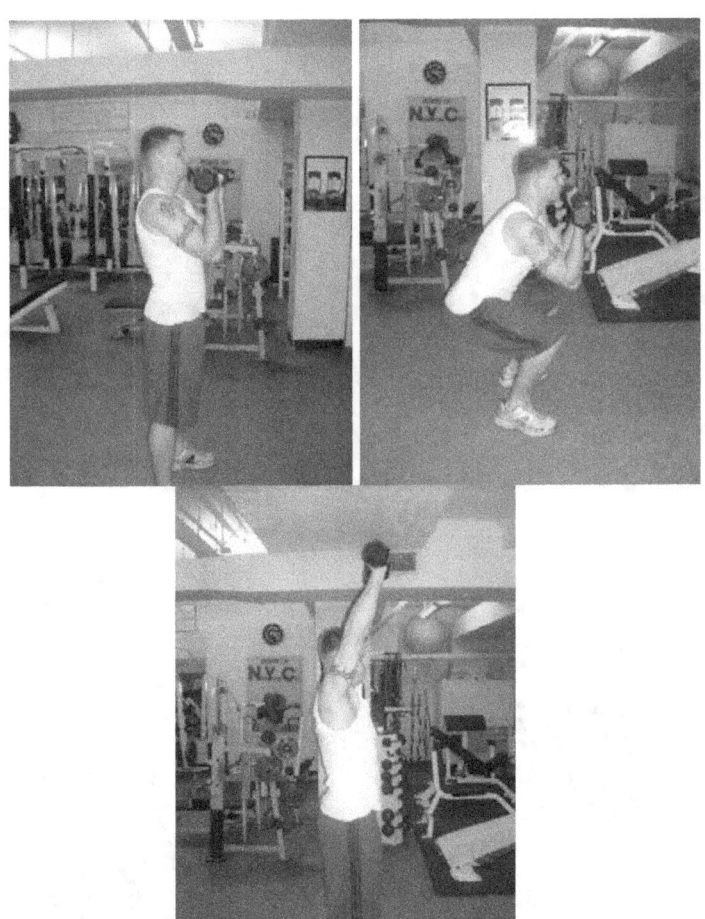

With the weights at shoulder level with palms facing your body, perform a regular squat.  On the way up using your arms and legs simultaneously, press the weight over your head finishing with palms facing away from you as seen in the photo. Use the same weight you would use on a regular Arnold press.

### 9.  Pullovers on ball

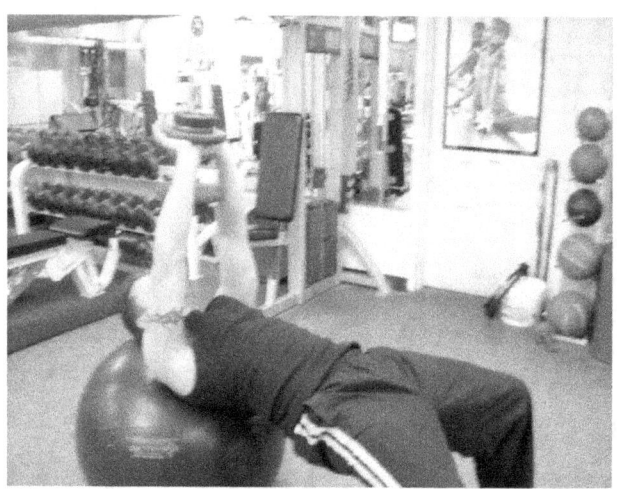

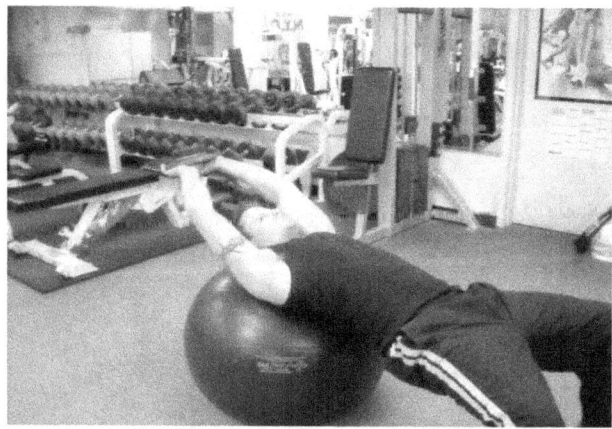

This is the same exercise that is done on a bench or floor. The ball adds a little balance and stability to the exercise and also brings your core into effect. Make sure your head and neck are resting on the ball. Do 10 reps.

## 10. Tricep Extension on ball

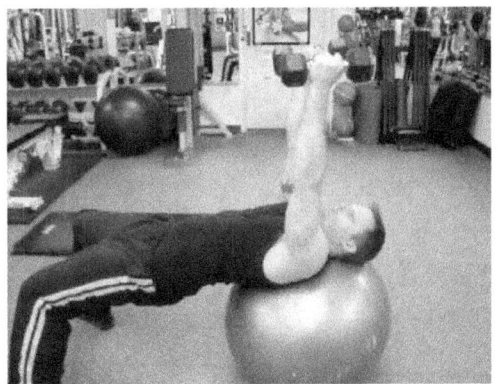

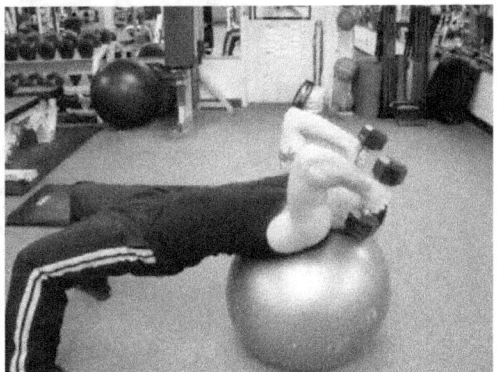

This is the same exercise done on the floor or bench. Use the same weight you would normally use on the tricep extension.

## 11. Stability ball crunch with weight

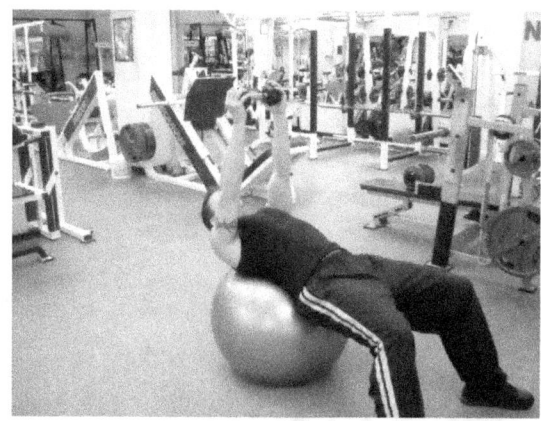

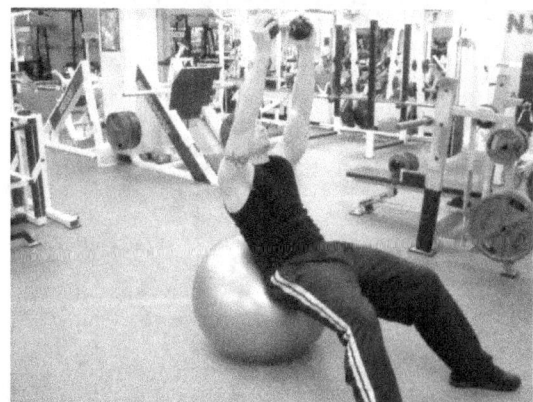

Get into position on the ball as shown in Photo 1.  Keeping your arms straight, lift the weight as high as you can using only your abdominal muscles. Use a weight heavy enough to perform 20-25 reps.

## 12. Walking Lunge

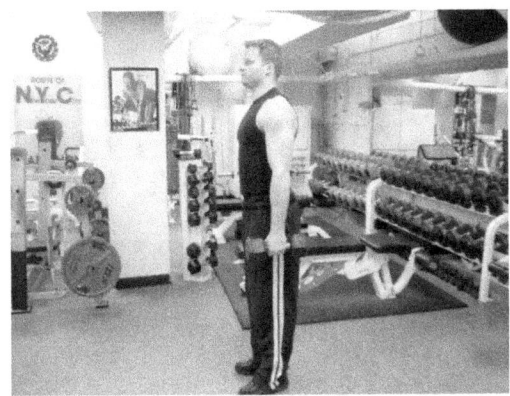

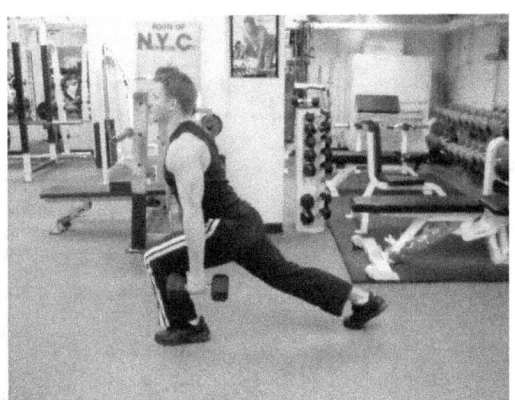

This is a variation of the regular lunge and is an exercise performed by athletes and anyone who wants to condition their body and work their legs at the same time. Use no weights when you first perform this exercise, working on your balance. Lunge with your left leg as seen in Photo 2. Go as low as possible then bring your right leg up to meet your left leg. Repeat with the opposite leg. Perform 10 reps each leg.

## 13. Plank Pushups

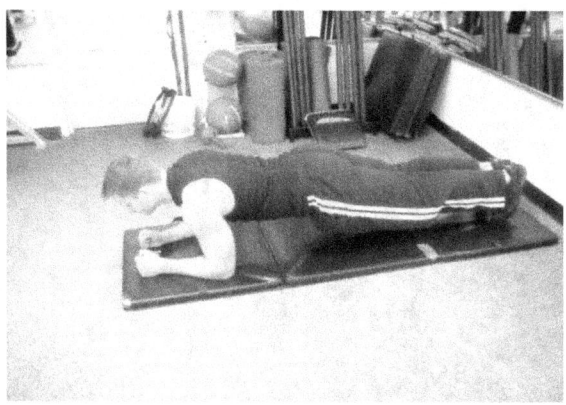

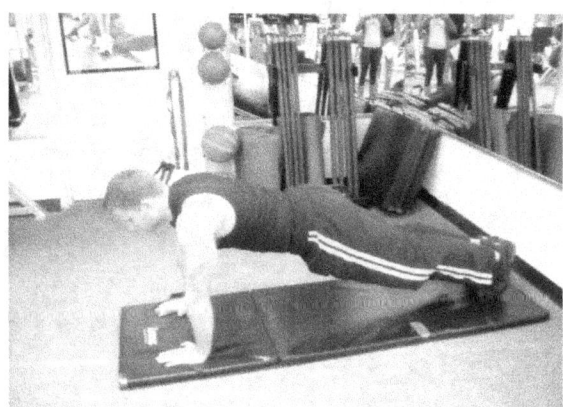

This exercise is great for your core as well as your triceps.  While in plank position, push up on to your hands, then return back to plank position and repeat.  Do 10 reps each arm.

## 14. Reverse fly on ball

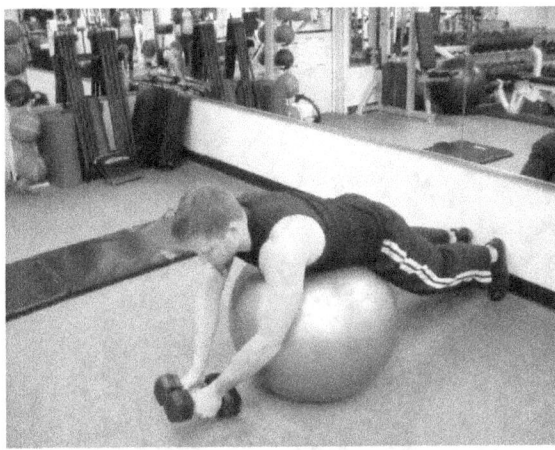

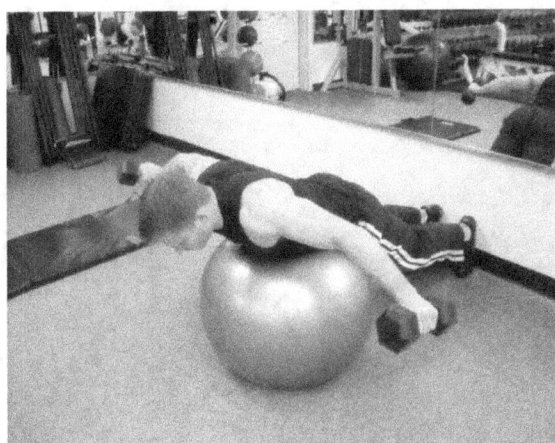

Lying face down on the stability ball with weights in front of you, perform the exercise the same as you would perform doing a bent over reverse fly.  Do 8-10 reps

## 15. Concentration Curl

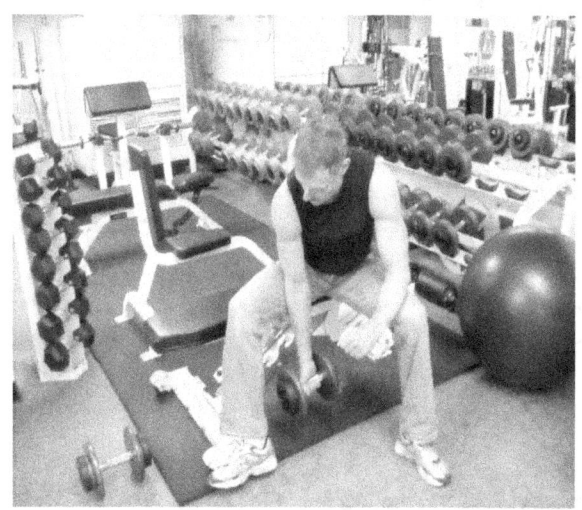

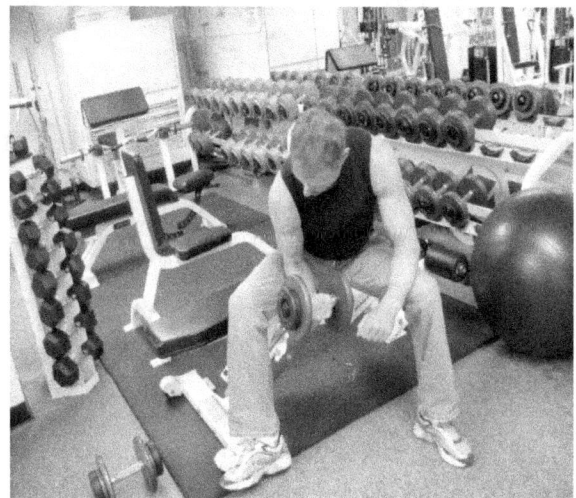

Sitting on a chair or bench, take a dumbbell and perform a bicep curl with your elbow on the inside of your leg.  Use a weight slightly lighter than your normal dumbbell curl.  Do 8 reps.

## The 2$^{nd}$ "C" Workout

The 2$^{nd}$ C workout can be done in the order that is written or you can take the exercises that you like and incorporate them into your other routines.  You also can take one exercise and perform it in as many sets as you like.  For example, if you just want to focus on legs you can take all the leg exercises and perform two or three sets of each.  If you want to work on upper body workouts you can do three or four sets each of the upper body movements. Any combination that you do is good. Remember for overall fitness the faster more intense workouts are the best.

"Exercise is habit forming – and it's a good habit to have
to improve your quality of life!"

## Final Thoughts

Being a fitness professional has been a rewarding and successful career for me. It not only enabled me to help all the clients and athletes that I've trained to achieve their goals, but has kept me in great shape as well. One of my clients asked me if I ever get tired of working out. My answer to that is, how can you get tired of doing something that makes you feel so good both mentally and physically? We all get tired of our everyday schedule sometimes. The same job, the same routine every day can get really boring but working out is an escape from all that.

Through the centuries people have been searching for the fountain of youth. Well let me tell you the only fountain of youth out there doesn't come in pill form. It's not in some secret location in a faraway place. The secret lies in your own mind. You find it when you decide to take charge of your life and your health. It comes from working out really hard with resistance exercise and hard cardio. From my experience in training people of all ages and abilities, observing their fitness state after years of training, my conclusion is that the harder you work the younger you will look and the fitter you will be as you age.

Working out hard makes a big difference in the way you age and people that do those hard workouts look much younger than their years and are much healthier than other people of the same age. My hard-working clients keep getting stronger year after year and don't have the joint problems or knee replacements that their peers have. The aging process can be prolonged, reversed, or halted, and my clients are a true testament to that. Thirty minutes of strength training and interval cardio workouts four to five times per week is the closest thing you will ever find to the fountain of youth.

What happens when older people stop their high intensity training? They regress very fast to being more like their real body age. One of my 75-year-old clients and her husband decided they didn't want to lift heavy weights anymore and would spend half the year on vacation without exercising. Well after a year they had their annual checkup and their doctor told them they had lost a good portion of their endurance and their bones showed signs of osteoporosis. Just part of growing old they said, however their doctor was smart enough to tell them it was a lack of exercise that caused it. Well after a year of getting back into the gym and lifting heavy weights again, they have gotten their stamina back and reversed the osteoporosis. Now they rarely miss a workout with me, knowing how important it is to maintain their optimum health by maintaining a regular workout schedule.

I've had other cases of people over 50 who get lazy so they stop coming to the gym. In every case there is a rapid muscle and bone density loss, weight gain, and loss of endurance. Someone in their 20's or 30's can stop working out for a month with little or no effect on their fitness level, however the older we get the faster our fitness level declines and the longer it takes to get it back. The good news is you can get back in shape faster than someone who has never worked out before because we all have something called "muscle memory". Our cells and muscles remember they were once in shape and can quickly respond to a renewed workout routine.

The bottom line is, if you aren't exercising now, start today! Once you start, never stop. If you follow those two rules, I guarantee the sky's the limit! You'll love how you feel with a Younger Body Now.

# Notes

1.  Blair, Steven N. HealthDay News;
www.nlm.nih.gov/medlineplus/print/news/fullstory/58437.html

2.  Link Between Physical Activity and Morbidity and Mortality;
Center for Disease Control; www.cdc.gov/nccdphp/sgr/mm.htm

3. Archer, Shirley, Strength Training Update, *American Fitness,*
1/19/2008

4.  Krane, Beth, UConn Advance, Exercise Scientist Recognized for
Research Accomplishments; 11/28/2006

5. Kraemer, William, Ph.D., Leg Workouts, *Men's Fitness*, October,
2003

6.  Singh, Dr. Maria Fiatarone, Exercise and Strength Training: It's
Never Too Late To Start, *Alliance for Aging Research*, Fall, 2001

7.  Mazzeo, Robert S. Ph. D., Exercise and Physical Activity for Older
Adults; *Medicine & Sports & Exercise*, Vol 30, #6, June, 1998

8.  Nelson, Mirian E., Ph.D., Physical Activity and Public Health in
Older Adults: Recommendation From the American College of Sports
Medicine and the American Heart Association; *Journal of the
American Hearth Association*, 8/1/2007

9. Physical Activity and Health: A Report of the Surgeon General,
Older Adults Fact Sheet, 11/17/1999,
www.cdc.gov.needphp/srg/olderad.htm

10. Strength Training Among Adults Aged >65 Years – United States, 2001, MMWR Weekly, 1/23/2004

11.  Kolata, Gina, Staying A Step Ahead of Aging, *New York Times*, 1/31/2008

12. Staying A Step Ahead of Aging, *Fort Mills Times*, 8/26/2009

13. If You Want To Age Gracefully, Lifelong Physical Activity Is A Must, www.preventdisease.com, 3/2008

14. How Exercise Improves Your Love Life, www.fitness.suite.101.com, 6/17/2007

15. Depression and Exercise, www.mayoclinic.com/health/depressionandexercise. 10/2007

16. Marano, Hara; Depression: A Good Workout, *Psychology Today*, 3/1/2004.

**For more information and news on upcoming products**

**Visit us on the Web at:**

**www.youngerbodybyart.com**